FODMAP COOKBOOK

FODMAP
MAGIC

Quick and Effortless Low-Fodmap Recipes to Relief
Symptoms of IBs and Gut Problems

GABRIELLA HOLLOWAY

Table of Contents

PART I

Chapter 1: Introduction to the Low FODMAP diet

Do you suffer from abdominal cramping and discomfort? If you spend your days feeling constipated, bloated, and feel the uncontrollable urge to use the bathroom? If so, you may suffer from IBS.

With so many diets on the market, it can be hard to decide which one is best for you! In the following chapters, you will be learning everything you need to know about the FODMAP diet and how it can benefit your life.

Unfortunately, there are several theories behind why individuals suffer from IBS. For many, there is 70% of women who suffer from IBS due to their hormones triggering the symptoms. As for others, the reasons could be anything from a sensitive colon, an immune response to stressors, sensitive brain activity in detecting gut contractions, or even a neurotransmitter serotonin being produced in the gut. While the doctors are unable to pinpoint an exact reason for IBS, the good news is that they are certain that IBS will not cause other gastrointestinal diseases and it is not cancer!

The right question to ask in this moment, is what can I do about it? We are here to tell you that the low FODMAP diet is the way to go. In the chapters to follow, you will learn everything from what the diet is, who the diet is for, what FODMAP even stands for, and why this diet will work for you. We cover the benefits of the diet and include an easy start guide so you can get rid of that discomfort and bloat as soon as possible!

To start, it is important to understand what the FODMAP diet is, and why it is something you need to start. However, before we start, here are some tips for the beginners who are just starting or considering the low FODMAP diet.

Getting Started

Before we begin, it is important to get a diagnosis from your family doctor. Many people self-diagnose themselves with IBS and place themselves on the low FODMAP diet. This is something we do not recommend. If you have symptoms such as pain and bloating, you should see a professional to rule out any possible life-threatening diseases.

What is IBS?

As mentioned, be sure to see a professional to attain an official prognosis of IBS. If you suspect you do have Irritable Bowel Syndrome, realize that you are not alone. In fact, around 15% of the population in the United States suffer from IBS symptoms. While the symptoms do vary from person to person, the typical symptoms are as follow:

- Bloating
- Constipation
- Diarrhea
- Lower Abdominal Pain
- Lower Abdominal Discomfort

If you suffer from any of these, it is important to consult with your doctor the specific symptoms you have. This will be vital as there are three different types of irritable bowel syndrome. These include:

- IBS with Constipation
  - Typically, IBS with constipation has symptoms including bloating, abnormally delayed bowel movements, stomach pains, and loose or lumpy stool.
- IBS with Diarrhea
  - Typically comes with symptoms including stomach pain, urgent need to use the bathroom, loose and watery stool
- IBS with alternating Diarrhea and Constipation

Due to the fact that there are several types of IBS, this makes it hard to determine a single drug treatment to help with the symptoms. As we mentioned earlier, you need to consult with a professional. Once you have done this and ruled out any other illnesses, it is time to take a look at your diet.

Who is the diet for?

Typically, the low FODMAP diet is meant for individuals suffering from IBS. The diet itself was created as one of the first food-based treatments to help relieve IBS symptoms. The good news is that up to 75% of patients who had IBS experienced symptom relief when they followed the low FODMAP diet. However, the diet is also helpful if you have any of the following:

- Digestive Disorder
  - Gastroesophageal Reflux Disease (GERD)
  - Crohn's Disease
  - Celiac Disease

- Vegan Gut
- Bloating

Once you have determined that the low FODMAP diet could help your symptoms, it is now time to learn what FODMAP even stands for! This is going to be vital information to carry with you through your diet so you understand what you are eating and why your body is reacting the way it does!

We understand that there are many different types of diets out there. Some of you may be wondering, can I follow my current diet and still follow the low FODMAP diet? The answer varies depending on which you follow, and we will try to answer in a simple manner:

- Vegetarian/ Vegan
  - Yes, this diet is more than possible to follow if you are vegan or vegetarian. With a few tweaks, you can find friendly options and still stick to your regular diet!
- Low-Salt
  - If you follow a low-salt diet, this diet is doable for you. However, it will be vital that you learn how to read and follow food labels. Luckily for you, this is information also included in this book!
- Gluten-Free
  - As you will be learning, the FODMAP diet does exclude wheat, which contains gluten. If you are gluten-free, this diet is easy to follow as you most likely will not be able to have it anyway!

- Kosher
  - o If you have to eat kosher, you can still follow this diet. It will be up to you to find certain kosher foods, but after the elimination diet, you will be able to find the foods and still stick to your original diet.

History of the low FODMAP diet

Originally, the low FODMAP diet was developed by a team of scientists at the Monash University located in Australia. The original research was meant to investigate if the diet would be able to control IBS symptoms with food alone. The university established a food analysis program to study FODMAPs in both Australian as well as international foods.

In 2005, the first FODMAP ideas would be published as part of a research paper. In the paper, the hypothesis was that by reducing dietary intake of certain foods that were deemed indigestible, this could help reduce symptoms stimulated in an individual's gut's nervous system.

Over many years, research has shown that certain short-chain carbohydrates such as lactose, sorbitol, and fructose was the cause behind gastrointestinal discomfort. Once the basis of digestion was studied, the low FODMAP diet was created to help with these symptoms.

What does FODMAP stand for?

FODMAPs are typically found in foods that we consume every day. They are in onions, rye, barley, wheat, garlic, milk, fruits, vegetables, and more! As you can tell from this very small list (don't worry, we will cover more in the chapters to follow), they are in some of our more common foods!

This is why it is so easy to feel bloated for some people, without understanding what is causing it! However, before we dive into how this diet works, you will need to understand the acronym FODMAP.

F-Fermentable

O- Oligosaccharies (short chain carbohydrates)

D- Disaccharides (lactose)

M- Monosaccharides (fructose)

A- and

P- Polyols (Sorbitol, xylitol, maltitol, and mannitol)

The reason you may be suffering from IBS or other digestive issues is due to the fact that most FODMAPs have a hard time absorbing into your small intestine. As a result, these FODMAPs are fermented by the bacteria in your small and large intestine in which results in bloating and irregular bowel movements.

While the FODMAPs cause the digestive discomfort, it is important to understand that it is not the cause of the intestinal inflammation itself. In fact, the FODMAPs produce alterations of intestinal flora that help you maintain a healthy colon. This does not change that the symptoms are still uncomfortable.

What may be causing your IBS symptoms could be a fructose malabsorption or a lactose intolerance. As you will be learning in later chapters, as you begin the low FODMAP diet, there will be an elimination phase where you learn what exactly is causing your symptoms and discomfort.

The source of the FODMAP will vary depending on different dietary groups. In more common circumstances they are compromised as the following:

- Oligosaccharies: Fructans and Galacto-oligosaccharies
- Disaccharies- Lactose
- Monosaccharies- Fructose
- Polyols- Xylitol, Mannitol, Sorbitol

Sources of Fructans

In later chapters, we will be going more in-depth on the foods you can and cannot eat. To cover the basics, you should understand where these specific irritants come from. To start, we will go over the source of fructans. These can be found in very popular ingredients including; rye, garlic, onion, wheat, beetroot, Brussel sprouts, and certain prebiotics.

Sources of Galactans

As for galactans, these are primarily found in beans and pulses. It can also be found in certain tofu and tempeh, but this does not mean that vegans and vegetarians cannot follow the low FODMAP diet. It simply means that you will need to find other sources of proteins if you want to follow a plant-based diet. We will be going over this more in the chapters to follow.

Sources of Polyols

Polyols are typically found in stone fruits. These include avocados, apples, blackberries, watermelon, and more. They are also found naturally in certain vegetables and bulk sweeteners.

While this diet may seem to be lacking many of your favorite foods, don't you worry! Due to the wide variety of IBS symptoms, it is unclear which foods trigger certain individuals. This is why the elimination trial will be important before you start the diet. Please remember that everyone is different. While some people see immediate results when they begin the diet, for others, it will take some time.

Effectiveness and Risks of the low FODMAP diet

It is important to understand that the low FODMAP diet is meant for short-term symptom relief. However, long-term diet can have a negative effect on your body. Unfortunately, it can be detrimental to your guy metabolome and microbiota. It is to be taken very seriously that this diet is meant for short periods of time and only under the advice of a professional.

Please understand that if you choose to follow the low FODMAP diet without any medical advice, it is possible the diet could lead to some serious health risks. Some of these risks are as followed:

- Nutritional Deficiencies

- Increased Risk of Cancer
- Death

When you start the low FODMAP diet, it is possible the diet itself could mask any serious disease that present themselves of digestive symptoms. These could include celiac disease, colon cancer, or inflammatory bowel disease. This is why it is so crucial to seek professional help before starting the diet on your own.

Now that you have learned the basics of the low FODMAP diet, it is time to learn all about the benefits that come with the diet change. Obviously, the main change will be to help lower any digestive troubles you may behaving. By removing the potential triggers in which are causing your digestive issues, this will help pinpoint which food intolerances you have.

While this diet may seem to take a lot of time and effort, think of the time you are wasting by being in discomfort all of the time and using the bathroom! With a few minor adjustments and tests, you will be able to find the source of your problem and hopefully never feel this way again! Now, onto learn all of the other incredible benefits the low FODMAP diet can bring to you!

Chapter 2: Benefits of the Low FODMAP diet

According to research, the low FODMAP diet is effective for around 75% of patients who suffer from IBS. In most cases, the patients are able reduce any major symptoms they are experiencing and in hand, improve their quality of life.

In the same research, scientist found evidence that the diet can also be beneficial for people who suffer from other functional gastrointestinal disorders such as Chron's disease, ulcerative colitis, and inflammatory bowel disease. All you need to do to benefit from this diet is to figure out what is causing the digestive disturbances and symptoms. Below, you will find some of the other benefits the low FODMAP diet has to offer:

A. IBS Symptom Reduction

By following the low FODMAP diet, individuals can reduce most symptoms involved with IBS including stomach pain, bloating, and gas. It is important to follow the diet and remove any irritants as they ferment inside of your intestines. By selecting foods that don't trigger your symptoms, you can avoid them altogether!

B. Chron's Disease Reduced Discomfort
By following the low FODMAP diet, individuals were able to change the quality and number of prebiotics. By controlling the foods you consume and avoiding the ones that trigger your system, you could reduce the discomfort you feel from the trigger foods.

C. Increased Energy

Some individuals feel tired no matter how much they eat through the day. It is believed that a low FODMAP diet can help reduce fatigue. This could be due to the fact that the body is no longer wasting energy on digesting foods that don't agree with your system. This is especially true for sweeteners that you could be using on a daily basis. As you will be learning later, some of the best sweeteners can be found in fruit!

D. Reduced Constipation and Diarrhea

When you follow the low FODMAP diet, you will begin to eliminate foods that are causing your symptoms in the first place. When you do this, your body will find a balance, and you may find that your bloating will decrease, the gas will decrease, and your stools will return to normal. It is a win-win situation! All you will need to do is figure out your triggers (which we cover in the third chapter) and follow the diet!

On top of these incredible benefits, there is also beliefs that the low FODMAP diet can benefit psychological health. Often times, the disturbances of IBS can cause stress to certain individuals, eventually leading to anxiety and depression. When you remove the trigger causing the symptoms by diet, you will be able to improve the quality of your life.

As you will be learning in the chapters to follow, the low FODMAP diet includes an elimination diet in order to get started. As you introduce foods, you may find that you have a lactose or gluten intolerance. While this may seem like a huge change, there are some incredible benefits to changing your diet.

Benefits of a Grain Free Diet

As you will be learning later in the book, there are many types of grains that has been found to cause inflammation. Unfortunately, this is a very common culprit for the digestive disorders you may be experiencing. This is especially true if you are very sensitive to gluten. The good news is that if you are looking to lose weight on top of feeling better, cutting out these grains will be the best thing to ever happen to you. Reined grains are high in carbohydrates and calories; they offer little to no nutrition and contribute to discomfort in your stomach. Before you make the switch to going grain free, consider some of the amazing benefits as follow:

A. Digestion Benefits

Gluten is a type of protein that can be found in wheat products. If you do the elimination diet and find that you are gluten sensitive, cutting it out makes the most sense. When you cut it out of your diet, this can help relieve issues such as nausea, bloating, diarrhea and constipation.

B. Reduced Inflammation

When you experience acute inflammation, this normally means that your immune system is fighting off foreign invaders. Unfortunately, if you sustain these levels for a long period of time, this is what causes chronic disease. By cutting gluten out, you can reduce the amount of inflammation in your body.

C. Balanced Microbiome

By following a grain-free diet, you will be able to balance the microbiome in your gut. When you do this, it helps support the beneficial bacteria in your body, helping improve your digestion, boost your immunity, and helps keep blood sugar under control.

D. Weight Loss

As mentioned earlier, most grains offer little to no nutrition. When you cut these extra calories out of your diet, it will help you lose weight. Instead of grains, try eating nutrient-dense foods like vegetables or legumes. Of course, you will figure out exactly what you can eat on the low FODMAP diet after going through the elimination portion.

Another common irritant when individuals suffer from IBS and other digestive orders can be lactose! You may be thinking to yourself; I could never give up my yogurt or ice cream. The good news is that in the current market, some incredible alternative choices can fit in the low FODMAP diet. In case you need some further benefits to help convince you, here are just a few:

E. Healthier Digestion

You may not know, but around 70% of the population has a degrees of intolerance to lactose. When we first begin to wean off of our mother's milk, we begin to use lactase. Lactase is an enzyme that helps digest lactose found in milk. As we age, we begin to lose the ability to digest lactose and is one of the biggest known triggers for IBS. By taking dairy out of your diet, you save yourself the troubles all together!

F. Decreased Bloating

Bloating occurs when we have issues with digestion. Some dairy products can cause excessive gas in the intestines, which is what causes the bloating in the first place. Some bodies are unable to break down the carbohydrates and sugar fully which in turn, creates an imbalance of gut bacteria.

G. Clearer Skin

If you suffer from acne, dairy could be the culprit! According to studies posted in Clinics in Dermatology, it was found that dairy products such as milk contain growth hormones that stimulate acne. By following the low FODMAP diet and cutting dairy from your diet, you could naturally treat acne!

H. Reduce Risk of Cancer

A 2001 study at Harvard School of Public Health found that there was a connection between high calcium intake and increased risk of prostate cancer. It is thought that the hormones in the milk contain contaminants such as pesticides that have been linked to cancer cell growth. These contaminants are mostly found in dairy products, giving you another reason to cut them from your diet altogether!

I. Decreased Oxidative Stress

It is believed that a high milk intake is typically associated with higher mortality rates in both men and women. This may be due to the D-galatose found in milk which helps influence oxidative stress and inflammation in the body. Unfortunately, this undesirable effect caused by milk can cause chronic expose and damage health. On top of inflammation, it can also shorten life spans, cause neurodegeneration and also decrease one's immune system.

As you can tell, there are so many incredible benefits of switching over to the low FODMAP diet. Whether you are looking to get rid of bloating, lose some weight, or stop constipation and/or diarrhea, the low FODMAP diet has got you covered. It is all a matter of figuring out what your trigger is in the first place.

Obviously, we could go on and on about the incredible benefits of the diet, but then we would never get to the diet itself! Now that you are aware of just some of the benefits, it is time to get you started! In the chapter to follow, you will be learning how to get started on the low FODMAP diet. You will the steps to get started on the diet itself and how to diet whether you are vegan, vegetarian, diabetics, or doing this for a child who suffers from IBS. When you are ready, we can dive in!

Chapter 3: Starting the Low FODMAP diet

Now that you are aware of the low FODMAP diet and some of its benefits, it is time to learn how you can get started on the diet yourself! While a diet and lifestyle change can seem daunting, it will be important to believe in yourself and remember why you started it in the first place. In the chapter to follow, we will be providing you with all of the information you need. From diagnosis of IBS, to starting the diet, and even how to practice if you are vegan, vegetarian, or diabetic. This diet can be universal; it is all about finding what works best for you. First, it is time to understand the diagnosis of IBS.

Getting Diagnosed with IBS and FODMAP Tests

If you are in the process of being diagnosed with a chronic medical condition, this could be a challenging time for you. It is important that you understand the symptoms the doctors are looking for, and which medical tests you will be taking in order to be officially diagnosed with irritable bowel syndrome. IBS can be diagnosed with a combination of Rome IV criteria so the doctors will be able to rule out any other gastrointestinal disorders.

Rome IV is a set of criteria that doctors have found that most IBS patients have in common. This criteria is 98% accurate when the doctors are identifying their patients with IBS. These criteria are as followed:

1. Recurrent abdominal pain at least one day per week in the last three months are have the following:

   A. Related to defecation

B. A change in stool frequency

C. Change in form of stool

2. Criteria from above is fulfilled with symptoms for at least six months before official diagnosis

Other symptoms often associated with IBS include bloating, abdominal pain, and a change in bowel habit. Your doctor will take in the evidence and match with the Rome IV criteria and will move onto discussing any red flag symptoms that may be occurring.

Before being diagnosed with IBS, it will be important that your doctor rules out any other medical conditions that could be presented with the same symptoms; this is where the red flag symptoms come into play. These flags include:

- Inflammatory Markers

- Rectal Masses

- Abdominal Masses

- Anemia

- Nocturnal Symptoms such as waking up from sleep to defecate

- Family History of coeliac disease, inflammatory bowel disease, and ovarian cancer

- Rectal Bleeding

- Unintentional Weight Loss

On top of these symptoms, your doctor will also ask for several other symptoms in order to diagnose you with IBS. Firstly, the discomfort and pain in your abdomen will need to be related to altered bowel frequency as well as a change in your stool form. You will also need to have at least two of the following symptoms:

1. Feeling incomplete emptying when using the bathroom
2. Passage of mucus when using the bathroom
3. Straining, Urgency, and Altered Stool passage
4. Abdominal Bloating
5. Lethargy
6. Backaches
7. Bladder Symptoms
8. Nausea

Medical Tests for IBS

Once your doctor figures out your symptoms, rules out any other serious medical conditions and believes it is appropriate to run tests for IBS can you expect one of the following tests:

- Antibody testing for coeliac disease
- C-reactive protein
- Erythrocyte sedimentation rate
- Full blood count

While these tests are typical, it may be different if you present any of the red flag symptoms from above. If you do have a red flag symptom, there will be additional tests to rule out any more serious issues. These tests are as follow:

- Hydrogen Breath Test (meant for lactose intolerance)
- Fecal Occult Blood

- Fecal Ova and Parasite Test

- Thyroid Function Test

- Rigid/ Flexible Sigmoidoscopy

- Ultrasound

In the case that your doctor feels your symptoms may not be linked to IBS, they will most likely refer you to a gastroenterologist. This is a physician who is an expert in managing diseases found in the liver and gastrointestinal tract. However, this is worst case scenario. For now, we will focus on following the diet if you are diagnosed with IBS.

Breaking down FODMAPS

In general, FODMAPs naturally occur in popular foods such as vegetables, fruits, grains, cereals, dairy products, and legumes. Unfortunately for those who suffer from IBS, these FODMAPs are absorbed poorly in our small intestines and can affect our bowels as a symptom. FODMAPs are short-chain carbohydrates found in these foods, but this does not mean that the diet itself is sugar-free. When we consume FODMAPs, they are fermented by gut bacteria in the large intestine in which triggers the unpleasant GI symptoms that you may be experiencing. Before we move onto the elimination stage, it is important to understand just what this acronym means.

Fermentable

Fermenting is the process where our gut bacteria attempt so break down FODMAPs. As you are already aware, these FODMAPs are indigestible carbohydrates and in turn, produce gas.

Oligo-Saccharies

This group of the FODMAP are broken down into two subgroups including fructans and galactans. Fructans also known as fructo-oligosaccharies or FOS are most commonly found in foods such as dried fruit, barley rye, wheat, garlic, onion. Galactans or galacto-oligosaccharies or GOS are found in pulses, legumes, cashews, pistachios, and silken tofu. If you feel yourself panicking over remembering these foods, don't worry. In the chapter to follow, we will cover exactly what you can and cannot eat while on the low FODMAP diet.

Di-Saccharies

As mentioned in the chapter from before, lactose could be a potential trigger in your diet. These can be found in any product that comes from goat, sheep, or cow's milk. Lactose itself contains two sugars united that require an enzyme known as lactase before our bodies are even able to absorb it. When your gut lacks these enzymes, this is when you can trigger symptoms of IBS.

Mono-Saccharides

This is a fructose that is found when a person has an excess amount of glucose in their diet. Our bodies need an equal amount of glucose in our system to stop any malabsorption. This means that while some of us can consume a certain amount of glucose, it is important to avoid foods that contain an excess amount. Some examples of these excessive foods include asparagus, honey, apples, and pears.

And Polyols

Polyols are also known as sugar alcohols. These can be found in a wide range of vegetables and fruits including sweet potatoes, mushrooms, pears, and apples. These sugar alcohols are also found artificial sweeteners in chewing gum, diabetic candy, and even protein powder. These polyols can only be partially absorbed into our small intestines. The rest continue into the large intestine, begin to ferment, and cause discomfort and bloating for some people.

As you begin to consider the low FODMAP diet, it is important to understand that one size does not fit all. This diet will change depending on your intolerance to certain foods. On the FODMAP diet, you will be following three different phases including: The Elimination Phase, The Reintroduction Phase, and the Maintenance Phase. We will go further into detail of each phase, so you have a full understanding before beginning.

The Elimination Phase

The Elimination phase is also known as the restriction phase. While this may seem intimidating, realize that this phase is only meant to last two to six weeks. This phase should only last long enough for you to gain control over your symptoms. Once this happens, you will move onto the reintroduction phase with the help of a professional. It is important that this stage is short as it can have long-term effects on your gut health.

To begin, you will want to create a personal list of foods you feel makes your IBS worse. If you are unsure which foods could be causing your symptoms, you will want to check out the next chapter to see an extended list of foods you should be avoiding. Some popular starters include chocolate, coffee, nuts, and certain fibers.

Once you have made your list, you will begin to eliminate these foods one at a time from your diet. It will take a couple of weeks before you notice any improvements. It does take some time for these foods to get through your system. However, if you do not notice any improvement, you will want to reintroduce these foods into your diet and try the next item on your list. Eventually, you will have a complete list of foods that trigger your IBS symptoms. Other popular foods to eliminate during this phase include: soy, gluten, and dairy products.

An important tool during this phase will be a food diary. This way, you will be able to keep track of which foods you are eating during the day, and any symptoms that may present themselves after they have been consumed. In general, the longer this phase is, the more likely you are to find that is triggering your IBS symptoms. It is important to remember that once eliminated, you will need to reintroduce foods slowly in the next phase.

The Reintroduction Phase

Once you have gone through your elimination period, you will be reintroducing these targeted foods back into your diet. While following the low FODMAP diet, you will need to introduce these foods back into your lifestyle one at a time.

As a tip for the reintroduction phase, we suggest starting on a Monday.

This way, you will be able to consume a small portion of the food, wait a few days, and see if you experience any symptoms. On day three, you can eat a larger portion and wait another couple days for any onset symptoms. Be sure to keep track of how you are feeling in your food diary so you can present it to a professional if need be. If you experience symptoms, this is a possible food trigger. If there is no symptom, you can assume that this certain food group is a good match for your diet.

After a while, you will have a complete list of foods that you need to assess, and you will start the elimination phase over again to double check. Once you eliminate and reintroduce, you will be able to create a diet you can stick with and eliminate any symptoms of IBS you may experience.

Maintenance Phase

While this may take time, the elimination and reintroduction phase are going to be very important while following the low FODMAP diet. These are going to be your tools in identifying foods that trigger your IBS symptom. The long-term goal is to create a wide variety of foods you can consume on a daily basis to ensure you are intaking all of your essential nutrients while eliminating the ones that make you feel lousy.

As you go through these phases, it is vital you listen to your body. Only you will be able to tell if you have a tolerance to certain foods. Remember that portion sizes will be important during these phases as well. While you may not react to small portions, larger portions may trigger the symptoms which you will want to avoid. The more tests you do, the more foods you will be able to add or subtract from your diet. While this may take some extra work, it will be worth it when you decrease your bloating and discomfort from IBS.

You may be wondering if you can follow this diet even if you have a certain lifestyle. Typically, the answer is yes! The only factor being that you could have a very limited number of foods allowed on your diet with any other limitations. Below, we will cover some of the more common diets and how you can also follow the low FODMAP diet as well!

Low FODMAP Diet with Vegan/Vegetarian Diet

If you follow a vegan or vegetarian diet, you may want to consider working with a dietary professional. Due to the fact you consume a diet that is different from most of the population, it can be more difficult to access foods that can work well with both diets. By working with a professional, they can ensure you still follow your diets without missing any essential nutrients your body needs.

While on the low FODMAP diet, it is important you keep re-testing foods. Remember that the elimination phase is meant to be short term. As you reintroduce old foods, you will be able to process if you can tolerate them or not. While you do this, you can find some staple foods, even if they happen to be high in FODMAPs.

If you follow a vegan or vegetarian diet, it will be vital that you pay special attention to your protein intake. As you will be learning later in the book, the low FODMAP diet includes a limitation of many legumes which may be a main source of protein for you right now. Instead of legumes, you can consider soy products or simply a smaller portion of legumes. Along with these switches, there are also milk substitutes to help with your protein intake. There is almond milk and other soy products to help out. Certain nuts and seeds also have varying levels of proteins for you to consider.

Low FODMAP Diet and Diabetes

If you have diabetes, you are most likely aware that there is no specific diabetic diet. In general, most people with diabetes follow a suggested balanced and healthy diet. If you wish to follow the low FODMAP diet while having diabetes, there are a few key rules you can follow to ensure you do not cause further harm to your health.

1. Planning

While on the low FODMAP diet, planning regular meals will be key. By doing this, you will be able to make sure that your blood glucose levels are always stable. By planning in advance, you can be successful in managing your diabetes while still following the low FODMAP diet. This stands especially true if you struggle finding healthy foods when you are away from your house. By being prepared, you will always have healthy options and can stay away from temptations. One good idea is to prep snacks for in-between your meals. These can be rice cakes, popcorn, or a simple fruit that is allowed in your low FODMAP diet.

2. Focus on Low FODMAP Carbohydrates

If you wish to follow the low FODMAP diet and eat healthy while having diabetes, eating starchy carbohydrates will be important for you. Some suitable options for you include wheat free bread, oats, potatoes, and rice. Before you include these, be sure to eliminate them from your diet to assure they are not triggers. Essentially, you will want to avoid any large portions of carbohydrates so you will be able to avoid any spikes in your blood glucose. You can do this by choosing slow-release carbohydrates like sweet potatoes or oats. On top of these carbs, you will also want to include allowed vegetables.

3.   High Sugar Foods

As a person with diabetes, you already know that sugary foods cause your blood glucose levels to rise. On the low FODMAP diet, there is a low risk of consuming sugary foods such as soft drinks and cake, but they should still be avoided.

4.   Low FODMAP Fruit

While fruits are a source of sugar, it will be important that you include a few portions of fruit per day. On the low FODMAP diet, there are plenty of options such as grapes, strawberries, bananas, and even oranges. You will want to pay special attention to your portion sizes as bigger portions, means higher amounts of fructose. You will also want to limit your portions of dried fruit, smoothies and fruit juices as they are typically pretty concentrated sources of fructose.

Low FODMAP Diet for Children

At this point, there has been very little research on the low FODMAP diet for children. Studies have shown that there are no real negative side effects for individuals who follow the low FODMAP diet for short period of time. However, if this diet were to carry on for longer than suggested, it could possibly have a negative effect on the gut flora balance in a child. If you are considering this diet for your child, there are several factors you will want to take into consideration.

First, your child will need to be seen by the pediatrician to confirm that your child has irritable bowel syndrome. Once it is diagnosed, the doctor will need to approve the diet and be carefully supervised to assure the safety of your child. Only after you follow these steps should you continue onto the elimination stage of the low FODMAP diet. For success on the diet, you can follow some of the following tips:

1. Inform Other Adults

Just like with any other diet restrictions, you will want to inform key adults of your child's restrictions. Whether it is a friend, a child care provider, or a teacher, this will be vital for the success of the diet. When these adults are in know of your child's diet, they will be able to address any stomach issues they may be having.

2. Involve Your Child

If your child is old enough, try to explain the diet to them in simple terms. You will want to explain that they are feeling sick due to the food they are eating. Be sure to include them and ask for their input in the food substitutions and menu. By making your child feel they are a part of the process, this may help your child comply with the new food rules.

3. Pack and Plan

Many parents fear diets for their children as they are always on the go! Luckily, the FODMAP diet is pretty easy to follow when you plan ahead. When you are at home, you most likely stock the fridge with low FODMAP foods. By planning ahead and packing your own snacks and lunches, you can assure your child will stick to the diet, so they do not make themselves sick.

4.   Forget the Small Stuff

Your kid is going to be a kid. If your child eats a restricted food every once in a while, it isn't going to ruin their diet altogether. Children typically do not have the self-discipline that adults have. They will most likely be tempted by restricted foods when at school or with their friends. You need to remember that while you want to stick to the diet most of the time, you can still allow your child some freedom when it comes down to what they are eating.

Exercise on the Low FODMAP Diet

While your diet may be causing your IBS symptoms, research has found that exercise can also help decrease any symptoms you may be suffering from. There are a few reasons why including regular moderate exercise will be important in the success of your diet.

First off, regular exercise can help reduce stress in your body. Typically, IBS tends to stress people out. When this happens, the nerves in your colon become tenser and can create abdominal pain. When your colon is tenser, this can slow down your bowel movements all together and cause constipation. A simple exercise such as cycling or walking can help release endorphins into your system and help release the tension in your colon. The more relaxed you are, the more flexible you will become.

Along with decreased stressed will come an increase of oxygen in your body. There are plenty of wonderful exercises such as tai chi and yoga that creates a breathing routine. When you take in these abdominal breaths, this helps increase the amount of oxygen in your body. As you increase oxygen, this will also help release any tension you are holding in your colon.

Finally, exercise can also increase your blood flow. As you begin to sweat, your body will be getting rid of toxins that could be creating discomfort in your colon. The more you sweat, the healthier you will be. Plus, the movement could help promote healthier bowel movements by moving blood to any problematic areas you may have.

As you consider exercise with your diet, remember that it will be vital to fuel your body before and after exercise. You will want to fuel about one to two hours before you work out. As long as it is included in your low FODMAP diet consider a banana with peanut butter or even oatmeal with some strawberries. The exercise can be any moderate activity of your choice from dancing, to running, to cycling, or even a little bit of strength training. Choose an exercise that makes you happy and one that you will stick with.

Reasons the Diet May Not Be Working

Speaking of sticking to a diet, some of you may follow these instructions and still suffer from IBS symptoms. If this still happens, you will want to take a look at your stress levels and the diet itself. While of course there is going to be a learning curve of the low FODMAP diet, allow yourself several weeks to change your food habits. Feel free to check back to the resources of this book to assure you are eating the foods allowed on the low FODMAP diet. If you still have no idea why you are experiencing the symptoms still, perhaps it is one of the following reasons that the diet isn't working:

1. Lack of Fiber

Fiber plays a very important role in keeping your stool regular. Often times, the low FODMAP diet will remove high fiber foods, which means you will need to pay special attention to your fiber intake. If you find yourself struggling, try speaking to a professional to find other options while on the low FODMAP diet. It will also be important that you drink plenty of water to move fiber through your system.

2. Too Much Fruit

While there are plenty of fruits on the low FODMAP diet, it is possible you are eating too much of it in one sitting. Typically, you will want to stick to only one serving at a time. If you want more fruit later in the day, try waiting two to three hours after the first one is consumed. As you practice this diet more, you will be able to tell your tolerance levels with the fruits so you can reduce that time in between servings.

3. Hidden FODMAPs

Often times, you could be consuming ingredients that are high in FODMAPs and have no idea. Typically, they are found in highly processed foods to help their taste and texture. FODMAPs are also found in some medications such as cough drops and cough syrup. Unfortunately, while they can help a cold, they are often high in sugar alcohols which can trigger your IBS symptoms. It will be important to read labels, which is included in the chapter to follow.

4. Portion Control

It is very easy to sit down and eat more than a portion. While on the low

FODMAP diet, allowed foods can become high FODMAPs when you exceed their allowed portion size. As an example, you may want to enjoy some rice cakes as a treat. A recommended serving size is only two rice cakes. If you eat double the allowed portion, this is when you may experience symptoms of IBS. Again, this is where reading labels carefully will come in handy while on the low FODMAP diet.

5. Stress

Stress is going to be a huge factor on the low FODMAP diet. If you are carefully following your diet, check your lifestyle. Stress itself can cause IBS symptoms so you may want to consider stress management skills along with a diet. You can try therapy or yoga. At the end of the day, your success is in your own hands.

If you continue to have IBS symptoms after following the diet and dealing with the issues from above, you may want to seek medical advice again. It is possible you have further intolerances that have not been explored yet. Also, the FODMAP diet will not work for everyone. If you have tried and failed, ask your doctor or dietician what the next step for you could be. For now, we will begin to cover the foods you can and cannot eat while on the low FODMAP diet.

Chapter 4: Low FODMAP diet foods

In the chapter to follow, you will find a list of both low and high FODMAP foods. As for the elimination phase, you will want to try to eliminate all of the high FODMAP foods. Once you are in the reintroduction stage, you will be able to introduce these foods back in order to see what is triggering your IBS symptoms.

As you choose your foods for your low FODMAP diet, remember that reading the ingredient list on a package is going to be vital for your diet success. Below, we will cover some of the basics of reading a food label. Too often, companies are able to hide food ingredients and could be triggering your symptoms without understanding why.

When you choose your foods, portion control will also be vital. When it comes to fruit, try your best to portion out one piece every few hours. As for processed foods, you will want to avoid them all together. If you ever have any doubts on low and high FODMAP foods, you can always revisit this chapter!

Reading and Understanding Nutrition Fact Label

If you are looking to eliminate certain foods from your diet, you will be surprised to learn that they can sneak into dishes without even realizing they are there. In order to stick with your diet, learning how to read and understand a nutrition fact label is going to be crucial for your diet.

A. Serving Size

When you first look at a label, you will want to check out the serving size along with the number of servings in any given package. These serving sizes are typically standardized so you can compare them to other similar foods. Remember that for some people, they can have smaller portions of FODMAP foods, but bigger portions could trigger IBS symptoms. When you are aware of a true serving size, this will make sticking to your diet a bit easier.

B. Calories

If you are on the low FODMAP diet to lose weight, this could be helpful for you. The calories in each package provide a measurement of how much energy comes in a serving of the food. The more calories you consume, the more you will gain weight. By being mindful of the calories in a portion, you will be able to manage your weight in a healthy manner.

C. Nutrients

When you look at a label, the first ones listed are typically the ones that Americans eat a good amount of. These can include Total Fat, Saturated Fat, Trans Fat, Cholesterol, and Sodium. While this isn't the main focus of the low FODMAP diet, it is something you should be mindful of for your general health.

D. Ingredients List

Finally, you will want to pay special attention to the ingredients list included on the package. If you are intolerant to certain ingredients, you will want to keep a food journal of these foods, so you always have them at hand to compare to a label. When looking at the ingredients list, they will be listed in order of weight from most to least. Eventually, you will know exactly what you can't eat and be able to compare easily in the store. As a beginner, remember to read the label of everything you put in your shopping cart.

When you understand the basics of reading a label, it is time to move onto learning the high and low FODMAP food list. We will begin with the high FODMAP foods. With this list, you will either want to avoid the foods altogether, or reduce them drastically. Of course, everyone's tolerances will be different but to help reduce any symptoms of IBS, you should reduce the following foods to enhance your health.

High FODMAP Foods (Avoid/ Reduce)

Fruits (High Fructose)

- Apples
- Avocado
- Apricots
- Blackcurrants
- Blackberries
- Boysenberry
- Currants
- Cherries
- Dates
- Figs
- Feijoa
- Guava
- Grapefruit
- Goji Berries
- Lychee
- Mango
- Nectarines
- Prunes
- Pomegranate
- Plums
- Pineapple
- Persimmon
- Pears
- Peaches
- Raisins
- Sultana
- Tamarillo
- Watermelon

Vegetables/ Legumes

- Asparagus
- Artichoke
- Butter Beans
- Broad Beans
- Black Eyed Peas
- Beetroot
- Bananas
- Baked Beans
- Choko
- Celery

- Cauliflower
- Cassava
- Fermented Cabbage
- Garlic
- Kidney Beans
- Leek
- Lima Beans
- Mushrooms
- Mixed Vegetables
- Pickled Vegetables
- Peas
- Red Kidney Beans
- Soy Beans
- Shallots
- Scallions
- Split Peas

Cereals and Grains

- Almond Meal
- Amaranth Flour
- Breadcrumbs
- Bread
- Biscuits
- Barley
- Bran Cereals
- Crumpets
- Croissants
- Cakes
- Cashews
- Cereal Bars
- Couscous
- Egg Noodles
- Freekeh
- Gnocchi
- Muesli Cereal
- Muffins
- Pastries
- Pasta
- Pistachios
- Udon Noodles
- Wheat Bran
- Wheat Cereals
- Wheat Flour
- Wheat Germ
- Wheat Noodles
- Wheat Rolls
- Spelt Flour

Sweeteners/ Condiments

- Agave
- Fruit Bar
- Fructose
- Hummus
- Honey
- High Fructose Corn Syrup
- Jam
- Molasses
- Pesto Sauce
- Relish
- Sugar-Free Sweeteners (Inulin, Isomalt, Lactitol, Maltitol, Mannitol, Sorbitol, Xylitol)
- Tahini Paste

Drinks

- Beer
- Coconut Water
- Fruit Juices (Apple, Pear, Mango)
- Kombucha
- Malted Drink
- Quinoa Milk
- Rum
- Soy Milk
- Soda
- Tea (Black Tea, Chai Tea, Dandelion Tea, Fennel Tea, Chamomile Tea, Herbal Tea, Oolong Tea)
- Whey Protein
- Wine

Dairy

- Cheese (Cream, Halloumi, Ricotta)
- Custard
- Cream

- Ice Cream/ Gelato

- Kefir

- Milk (Cow, Goat, Evaporated Milk, Sheep)

- Sour Cream

- Yogurt

While this may seem like a large list of foods you shouldn't eat, remember that ingredients will affect individuals a little differently. While you should limit the foods listed from above, it is okay to have them every once in a while. The point of this diet is to help reduce symptoms from IBS and bloating. At the end of the day, you are in charge of what you eat and understand how certain foods will make you feel.

Low FODMAP Foods

Fruits

- Ackee
- Breadfruit
- Blueberries
- Bilberries
- Bananas (Unripe)
- Clementine
- Cranberry
- Cantaloupe
- Carambola
- Dragon Fruit
- Guava (Ripe)
- Grapes
- Honeydew
- Kiwi Fruit
- Lime
- Lemon
- Mandarin
- Orange
- Plantain
- Papaya
- Passion Fruit
- Rhubarb
- Raspberry
- Strawberry
- Tangelo
- Tamarind

Vegetables

- Alfalfa
- Butternut Squash
- Brussel Sprouts
- Broccolini
- Broccoli
- Bok Choy
- Beetroot
- Bean Sprouts
- Bamboo Shoots
- Cucumber
- Courgette
- Corn

- Choy Sum
- Cho Cho
- Chives
- Chili
- Chick Peas
- Celery
- Carrots
- Cabbage
- Eggplant
- Fennel
- Ginger
- Green Pepper
- Green Beans
- Kale
- Leek Leaves
- Lentils
- Lettuce
- Olives
- Okra

- Pumpkin
- Peas (Snow)
- Parsnip
- Red Peppers
- Radish
- Sweet Potato
- Swiss Chard
- Sun-Dried Tomatoes
- Squash
- Spinach
- Spaghetti Squash
- Seaweed
- Scallions
- Turnip
- Tomato
- Water Chestnuts
- Yams
- Zucchin

Meat and Poultry

- Beef
- Chicken
- Deli Meats
- Lamb

- Prosciutto
- Pork
- Turkey
- Processed Meats

Seafood and Fish

- **Fresh Fish (Cod, Haddock, Salmon, Trout, Tuna, Canned Tuna)**

- **Seafood (Crab, Lobster, Mussels, Oysters, Shrimp)**

Breads, Cereals, Grains, and Nuts

- Bread
  Wheat Free
  Gluten Free
  Potato Flour
  Spelt Sourdough
  Rice
  Oat
  Corn
- Pasta
  Wheat Free
  Gluten Free
- Almonds
- Biscuit (Shortbread)
- Buckwheat (Noodles, Flour)
- Brazil Nuts
- Brown Rice
- Crackers

- Corn Tortillas
- Coconut Milk
- Cornflakes
- Corncakes
- Crispbread
- Corn Flour
- Chips (Plain)
- Mixed Nuts
- Millet
- Macadamia Nuts
- Oatcakes
- Oats
- Oatmeal
- Pretzels
- Potato Flour
- Popcorn
- Polenta

- Pine Nuts
- Pecans
- Rice
  White
  Rice
  Brown
  Basmati
- Rice Krispies
- Rice Flour
- Rice Crackers

- Rice Cakes
- Rice Bran
- Seeds
  Sunflower
  Sesame
  Pumpkin
  Poppy
  Chai
- Tortilla Chips
- Walnuts

Condiments, Sweets, and Sweeteners

- Almond Butter
- Acesulfame K
- Aspartame
- Chocolate
  White
  Milk
  Dark
- Erythritol
- Fish Sauce
- Glycerol
- Glucose
- Golden Syrup
- Jelly

- Ketchup
- Mustard
- Miso Paste
- Mayonnaise
- Marmite
- Marmalade
- Maple Syrup
- Oyster Sauce
- Peanut Butter
- Rice Malt Syrup
- Sucralose (Sugar)
- Stevia

- Sweet and Sour Sauce
- Shrimp Paste
- Saccharine
- Tomato Sauce
- Tamarind
- Vinegar
  Rice Wine Vinegar
  Balsamic Vinegar
  Apple Cider Vinegar
- Worcestershire Sauce
- Wasabi

Drinks

- Alcohol (Wine, Whiskey, Gin, Vodka, Beer)
- Coffee
- Chocolate Powder
- Protein Powder (Whey, Rice, Pea, Egg)
- Soya Milk
- Sugar-Free Soft Drinks
- Water

Dairy/ Eggs

- Butter
- Cheese (Swiss, Ricotta, Parmesan, Mozzarella, Goat, Fetta, Cottage, Cheddar, Camembert, Brie)
- Eggs
- Milk (Rice, Oat, Macadamia, Lactose-free, Hemp, Almond)
- Swiss Cheese
- Soy Protein
- Sorbet
- Tofu
- Tempeh
- Yogurt (Goat, Lactose-free, Greek, Coconut)

Herbs and Spices

- Bay Leaves
- Basil
- Curry Leaves
- Coriander
- Cilantro
- Fenugreek
- Lemongrass
- Mint
- Oregano
- Parsley
- Rosemary
- Sage
- Thyme
- Tarragon
- All Spice
- Black Pepper
- Chili Powder
- Cardamom
- Curry Powder
- Cumin
- Cloves
- Five Spice
- Fennel Seeds

- Nutmeg
- Saffron
- Turmeric
- Avocado Oil
- Coconut Oil
- Canola Oil
- Olive Oil
- Sesame Oil
- Sunflower Oil
- Soy Bean Oil
- Vegetable Oil
- Baking Soda
- Baking Powder
- Cocoa Powder
- Ghee
- Gelatin
- Lard
- Salt
- Yeast

As you can tell from the list from above, there are food choices for all different types of diets. Whether you are vegan, vegetarian, or follow a typical diet, there are plenty of choices for you.

The list from above may seem daunting, but as you learn your own version of the low FODMAP diet, you will be able to put together recipes from the ingredients you are allowed. The key to being successful on this diet is enjoying the foods you are allowed. Luckily in today's market, there are plenty of substitutes for ingredients that may trigger you. As long as you take the time to make this list, you will be able to make your new diet successful.

In the chapter to follow, we will be providing a couple different meal plans for you to follow. There will be a seven-day example vegan diet. Once you have read through this, you can move onto the fourteen-day low FODMAP starter diet. Remember that these are mere suggestions and you can make adjustments as needed.

Chapter 5: Low FODMAP Diet Meal plan

At this point in the book, you hopefully have a better understanding of the foods you can and cannot eat while on the low FODMAP diet. Before we jump into potential meal plans for you to follow, it is time to learn some delicious ingredients.

If you feel nervous about the diet due to the big list of foods to avoid, you absolutely shouldn't! Is your diet going to be different? Yes. However, when you are no longer experiencing diarrhea, constipation, bloating, and the other symptoms from IBS, you will be asking yourself why you didn't start sooner!

As you will find out from the recipes from below, there is a way to stick to your diet and enjoy your meal at the same time. You will find easy to make breakfast, lunch, and dinner recipes. Remember to pay special attention to the ingredients so you can determine if the recipe itself will stick within your own limits.

Low FODMAP Breakfast Recipes:

Small Banana Pancakes

Prep Time: Five Minutes

Cook Time: Twenty Minutes

Servings: Two

Portion: Four Mini Pancakes

Ingredients:

- Dairy-free Spread (Olive Oil) (3 T.)
- Ground Nutmeg (.25 t.)
- Ground Cinnamon (.50 t.)
- Salt (.125 t.)
- Baking Powder (.25 t.)
- Brown Sugar (1 T.)
- Gluten-free All-Purpose Flour (2 T.)
- Egg (2)
- Banana (2 Small, Unripe)

Instructions

1. Begin by heating a medium pan over medium heat before tossing in your dairy-free spread.
2. While this is cooking, go ahead and peel the banana before placing it into a bowl. Mash the banana until it becomes smooth and then add in the egg.
3. Once the egg and banana are mixed well, go ahead and add in the rest of the ingredients. At this point, you should have a mixture that resembles batter.
4. Spoon the mixture into your heated pan and cook the pancakes for a few minutes on each side or until they turn a nice golden color.
5. For extra flavor, try topping the pancakes with your favorite low FODMAP fruit!

Roasted Sausage and Vegetable Breakfast Casserole

Prep Time: Twenty-Five Minutes

Cook Time: Forty-Five Minutes

Servings: Eight

Ingredients:

- Eggs (12)
- Low FODMAP Milk (.50 C.)
- Dried Oregano (.50 t.)
- Salt and Pepper (.25 t.)
- Leek Tips (.50 C.)
- Red Bell Pepper (1)
- Lamb Sausage (1 Package)
- Baby Spinach (2 C.)
- Potato (1)
- Butternut Squash (1)
- Sweet Potato (1)
- Olive Oil (1 T.)

Instructions:

1. Before you begin prepping your food, you will want to preheat your oven to 400 degrees.
2. As your oven heats up, prepare the vegetables from the list above by peeling them and dicing the ingredients into bite-size pieces.

3. Once this is done, place the vegetables on a tray and drizzle them lightly with olive oil or a spread that is allowed on your own low FODMAP diet. Pop them into the heated oven for twenty minutes or until they are soft.

4. While the vegetables are cooking, you can cook your red bell pepper, leek, and sausage in a pan over medium heat. Be sure to cook all of these ingredients through.

5. Now that all of these ingredients are cooked, add in the vegetables to a large casserole dish.

6. In a small bowl, mix together the eggs and add in desired spices. When ready, gently pour the mix over the vegetables already placed in the casserole dish.

7. Place the dish in the oven for thirty minutes or until the eggs are set. This is a great dish to enjoy hot or cold for breakfast!

Blueberry Low FODMAP Smoothie

Prep Time: Five Minutes

Servings: One

Ingredients:

- Lemon Juice (1 t.)
- Maple Syrup (.50 T.)
- Rice Protein Powder (2 t.)
- Frozen Banana (1)
- Ice Cubes (6-10)
- Blueberries (20)
- Vanilla Soy Ice cream (.25 C.)
- Low FODMAP Milk (.50 C.)

Instructions:

1. Place all of the ingredients from above into a blender. Be sure to cut the frozen banana into smaller pieces.
2. Serve right away for a delicious breakfast.

Banana and Oats FODMAP Breakfast Smoothie

Prep Time: Five Minutes

Servings: One

Ingredients:

- Almond Milk (.50 C.)
- Linseeds (1 t.)
- Rolled Oats (1 T.)
- Banana (1)

Instructions:

1. Place all of the ingredients from above into a blender. Be sure you cut the banana into smaller pieces for easier blending.
2. Serve immediately for a filling and healthy meal.

Blueberry, Banana, and Peanut Butter Breakfast Smoothie

Prep Time: Five Minutes

Servings: One

Ingredients:

- Ice Cubes (6-10)
- Low FODMAP Milk (.75 C.)
- Blueberries (.50 C.)
- Peanut Butter (1 T.)
- Banana (.50)

Instructions:

1. Place all of the ingredients from above into a blender and blend until everything is smooth.
2. Serve immediately and enjoy!

Kale, Ginger, and Pineapple Breakfast Smoothie

Prep Time: Five Minutes

Servings: One

Ingredients:

- Ice (1 C.)
- Ginger (.25 T.)
- Kale (1 C.)
- Pineapple (.75 C.)
- Orange (.50)
- Low FODMAP Milk (1 C.)

Instructions:

1. Place all of the ingredients from above into a blender and blend until everything becomes smooth.
2. Serve immediately for a nice, healthy breakfast.

Strawberry and Banana Breakfast Smoothie

Prep: Five Minutes

Servings: One

Ingredients:

- Ice (1 C.)
- Maple Syrup (1 t.)
- Low FODMAP Milk (.75 C.)
- Strawberries (6)
- Banana (1)

Instructions:

1. Toss all of the ingredients into your blender and mix together until smooth.
2. Serve and for an extra treat, try adding some whipped cream!

Low FODMAP Soups and Salads:

Apple, Carrot, and Kale Salad

Prep Time: Ten Minute

Servings: Eight

Portion: .50 C.

Ingredients:

- Salt and Pepper (.25 t.)
- Maple Syrup (1.50 t.)
- Mustard (1 T.)
- Red Wine Vinegar (1.50 T.)
- Olive Oil (3 T.)
- Kale (.50 C.)
- Carrots (3)
- Apple (1 C.)

Instructions:

1. First step, you will want to create your dressing for the salad. You can do this by taking a small bowl and mixing together the maple syrup, mustard, vinegar, and oil. For some extra flavor, season with salt and pepper to taste.
2. Once this is done, take the kale, carrots, and apple and chop into fine, smaller pieces.
3. Finally, dress the salad, toss it a bit, and your meal is ready to be served!

Green Bean, Tomato, and Chicken Salad

Prep Time: Fifteen Minutes

Servings: Four

Portion: .50 C.

Ingredients:

- Lettuce (1 C.)
- Basil Leaves (2 T.)
- Cherry Tomatoes (10)
- Gruyere Cheese (.50 C.)
- Cooked Chicken (1 Lb.)
- Green Beans (.50 C.)

Instructions:

1. To begin, you will want to bring a medium pot of water to a boil. Once the water is boiling, cook your green beans for a few minutes. Once they are tender, drain the water from the pot and run the beans under cold water for a minute.

2. Next, take a large bowl and mix together all of the ingredients from above for a healthy salad.

3. For extra flavor, top your salad with any low FODMAP approved dressings.

Tuna Salad Low FODMAP Style

Prep Time: Five Minutes

Servings: Six

Portion: .50 C.

Ingredients:

- Salt and Pepper (to taste)
- Dried Dill (.50 t.)
- Lemon Juice (1.50 T.)
- Mayonnaise (.50 C.)
- Celery (.50)
- Tuna (2 Cans)

Instructions:

1. Start out by squeezing the liquid out of the tuna.
2. Once you have discarded the tuna, add it into a medium bowl with the vegetables from above.
3. When everything is stirred together, add in the dill, lemon juice, mayonnaise, along with the salt and pepper.
4. This mixture is great for any salad or sandwich!

Low FODMAP Pumpkin Soup

Prep Time: Ten Minutes

Cook Time: Fifteen Minutes

Servings: Six

Portion: 1 C.

Ingredients:

- Lactose-free Half and Half (.75 C.)
- Light Brown Sugar (1 T.)
- Canned Pure Pumpkin (1)
- Vegetable Soup Base (2 T.)
- Water (3 C.)
- Cayenne Pepper (.125 t.)
- Nutmeg (.25 t.)
- Cinnamon (.25 t.)
- Smoked Paprika (.25 t.)
- Scallions (.75 C.)
- Olive Oil (1 T.)
- Unsalted Butter (2 T.)
- Salt and Pepper to taste

Instructions:

1. To begin, you will want to heat up a medium sized pot over a low to medium heat. Once the pot is warm, you can add in your oil and butter until it begins to sizzle.

2. When the butter and oil are warm, add in your spices with the scallions and cook until they are soft.

3. Once this happens, add in the soup and water. Be sure to mix everything together before you add in the salt, brown sugar, and the canned pumpkin.

4. Now that these ingredients are placed in the pot, lower your heat and allow these to simmer for ten minutes or so. Feel free to stir every once in a while, to assure the ingredients are blended well.

5. Now, remove the soup from the heat and add in your half and half. Once the soup is cool, you can place the mixture into a blender and blend until it is smooth.

6. For extra flavor, season the soup with salt and pepper to taste.

Quinoa and Turkey Meatball Soup

Prep Time: Fifteen Minutes

Cook Time: Twenty Minutes

Servings: Eight

Portion: 1 C.

Ingredients:

- Collard Greens (5 C.)
- Celery (.50)
- Leek Tips (1 C.)
- Olive Oil (2 T.)
- Egg (1)
- Dried Basil (2 T.)
- Parsley (2 T.)
- Cooked Quinoa (.50 C.)
- Ground Turkey (1 Lb.)
- Turkey Stock (10 C.)
- Salt and Pepper to taste

Instructions:

1. To start out, you are going to want to make your meatballs for the soup. You will do this by taking a large mixing bowl and combine the egg, parsley, basil, quinoa, and turkey together. Gently take the mixture in your hands and form one inch balls.

2. Next, take a medium pan over medium heat and cook the turkey meatballs in olive oil for a few minutes. Be sure to flip the balls over so that they are a nice golden-brown color all around.

3. Now that these are done, take a large pot over medium heat and add in a tablespoon of oil. Once the oil is sizzling, you can add in the leek and celery. Sauté these two ingredients for a minute before adding in the collard greens and stock.

4. When all of the ingredients are cooked, add in the meatballs and allow this mixture to simmer over a low heat for eight to ten minutes.

5. Remove the soup from the heat and allow to cool slightly before serving.

Mixed Vegetable, Bean and Pasta Soup

Prep Time: Fifteen Minutes

Cook Time: Thirty Minutes

Servings: Fourteen

Portion: .75 C.

Ingredients:

- Gluten-free Pasta (1 C.)
- Dried Thyme (1 t.)
- Smoked Paprika (1 t.)
- Dried Basil (1 t.)
- Zucchini (1)
- Squash (1)
- Bok Choy (2 C.)
- Carrots (3)
- Kale (1 C.)
- Red Potatoes (1 C.)
- Butternut Squash (1 C.)
- Crushed Tomatoes (1 Can)
- Water (8 C.)
- Leek Tips (.25 C.)
- Scallions (.75 C.)
- Olive Oil (2 T.)
- Salt and Pepper to taste

Instructions:

1. To start, you will want to take a large pot and begin to heat it over medium heat with the olive oil placed in the bottom.

2. Once the olive oil is sizzling, add in the leeks and scallions and allow them to cook until they become soft.

3. When these are ready, add in your prepared zucchini, squash, Bok choy, carrots, kale, potatoes, chickpeas, canned tomatoes, and the water. Season as desired and place the top on the pot.

4. Bring all of the ingredients from above to a boil and then turn the heat down to allow everything to simmer for at least thirty minutes. By the end, all of the vegetables should be tender.

5. While the soup cooks, you can cook the gluten-free pasta in another pot so by the end, you can combine everything and have a healthy meal!

Vegan Options:

Low FODMAP Coconut and Banana Breakfast Cookie

Prep Time: Ten Minutes

Cook Time: Twenty Minutes

Servings: Ten

Portion: One

Ingredients:

- Vanilla Extract (1 t.)
- Vegetable Oil (.25 C.)
- Maple Syrup (.25 C.)
- Banana (1)
- Baking Powder (.50 t.)
- Cinnamon (1 t.)
- Ground Flax Seeds (2 T.)
- Chia Seeds (2 T.)
- Unsweetened Coconut Flakes (.50 C.)
- Banana Chips (.50 C.)
- Gluten-free All-purpose Flour (.50 C.)
- Old-fashioned Oats (1 C.)

Instructions:

1. You will want to begin by heating your oven to 325 degrees.

2. While the oven heats up, take a medium bowl and mix together the baking powder, cinnamon, flax seeds, chia seeds, coconut flakes, banana chips, flour, and oats altogether.

3. In another bowl, mix together a mashed banana, vanilla, vegetable oil, and pale syrup. When both bowls are well combined, you can mix them together and begin to create your dough.

4. Next, take a greased cookie sheet and lay out balls of dough to create your cookies. When this is done, pop the cookie sheet in the oven for twenty minutes.

5. When the time is up, remove the cookies, allow to cool, and enjoy!

Lemon and Garlic Roasted Zucchini

Prep Time: Five Minutes

Cook Time: Twenty Minutes

Servings: Twelve

Portion: 1 C.

Ingredients:

- Olive Oil (1.50 T.)
- Zucchini (2)
- Lemon Zest (2 T.)
- Salt and Pepper to taste

Instructions:

1. You can begin by heating your oven to 425 degrees.
2. While this warms up, slice your zucchini into thin slices and place in a bowl with the lemon zest and olive oil. Assure it is covered completely before seasoning with salt and pepper.
3. Place the zucchini on a greased sheet pan and cook for twenty minutes.

Rainbow Low FODMAP Slaw

Prep Time: Ten Minutes

Servings: Twenty

Portion: 1 C.

Ingredients:

- Pomegranate Seeds (.50 C.)
- Carrots (3)
- Kale (1 C.)
- Red Cabbage (1 C.)
- Green Cabbage (1 C.)
- Lactose-free Yogurt (.50 C.)
- Dijon Mustard (1 t.)
- Sugar (2 T.)
- Apple Cider Vinegar (.25 C.)
- Canola Oil (.50 C.)

Ingredients:

1. Start out by creating your dressing for the slaw. You can do this in a small bowl, mix together the canola oil, apple cider vinegar, Dijon mustard, sugar, yogurt, and a little bit of salt.
2. In another bowl, toss together the different cabbage with the carrots and the kale.
3. Gently drizzle the dressing over the kale, and you have a delicious slaw that is full of color and flavor!

Vegan Roasted Red Pepper Farfalle

Prep Time: Ten Minutes

Cook Time: Ten Minutes

Servings: Four

Portion: 1 C.

Ingredients:

- Capers (.25 C.)
- Parsley (.75 C.)
- Olive Oil (.25 C.)
- Roasted Red Peppers (1 Jar)
- Gluten-free Farfalle Pasta (2 C.)

Instructions:

1. You can start this recipe by cooking your pasta according to the instructions on the side of the box.
2. Once the pasta is cooked through, drain the water and then place the pasta back into the pot.
3. Toss in the oil, parsley, roasted red peppers, and capers to the mixture.
4. Mix everything together and season with salt and pepper for extra flavor.

As you can tell, you can follow the low FODMAP diet and still enjoy delicious foods. While these are only some of the many recipes you can follow on your diet, there are plenty of resources out there to provide you with even more! With these resources in hand, we will now go over a simple seven and fourteen-day meal plan that is easy to follow.

With a limited food choices, you may be thinking to yourself that you are going to get bored quick. When it comes to a new diet, it is all about your frame of mind. On one hand, you could think negatively about it and return to your old eating habits. With choice, comes consequence. When you eat the foods that trigger you, you are going to feel lousy. Why make that choice when you can choose to eat healthy and feel better? Below, we will provide some simple meals for you to consider until you feel confident enough to create your own recipes

Breakfast Meal Plan Ideas:

- Eggs- Hard-boiled, over easy, or even scrambled. There are many ways to enjoy eggs!
- Lactose-Free Yogurt with any low FODMAP fruit
- Gluten-free Muffins
- Gluten-free French toast
- Gluten-free Oatmeal with cinnamon
- Rice Cereal with low FODMAP fruit
- Ground Turkey
- Smoothie with low FODMAP fruit

Lunch Meal Plan Ideas:

- Gluten-free Bread with Deli Meat and Cheese

- Chicken Noodle Soup
- Quinoa Bowl with low FODMAP Veggies or Grilled Chicken
- Salad
- Baked Potato with Lactose-free Butter

Dinner Meal Plan Ideas:

- Stir-Fried Rice
- Tacos
- Gluten-Free Pizza
- Grilled Chicken Salad
- Steak with Fresh Low FODMAP Vegetables
- Grilled Chicken with White Rice
- Rice Pasta with Marinara
- Snack Meal Plan Ideas:
- Rice Cakes with Peanut Butter
- Baby Carrots
- Lactose-free Yogurt
- Unripe Banana
- Unsalted Peanuts
- Pop Chips
- Gluten-free Pretzels
- Crackers with Cheese
- Hard-Boiled Egg

14- Day Meal Plan

Week One:

Meal	Monday	Tues.	Wed.	Thurs.	Friday
BFast	Small Banana Pancakes	Blueberry Smoothie	Roasted Sausage and Vegetable Breakfast Casserole	Strawberry and Banana Breakfast Smoothie	Banana and Oats FODMAP Breakfast Smoothie
Lunch	Apple, Carrot, and Kale Salad	Mixed Vegetable, Bean, and Pasta Soup	Low FODMAP Pumpkin Soup	Tuna Salad Low FODMAP Style	Quinoa and Turkey Meatball Soup
Dinner	Low FODMAP Veggie Latkes	Steak with Lemon and Garlic Roasted Zucchini	Left Over Mixed Vegetable, Bean, and Pasta Soup	Vegan Roasted Red Pepper Farfalle	Salad with Grilled Chicken and Homemade Dressing

Meal	Saturday	Sunday
Breakfast	Eggs and low FODMAP fruit	Rice Cereal with low FODMAP fruit
Lunch	Chicken Noodle Soup	Baked Potato with Lactose-free Butter
Dinner	Stir-Fried Rice	Gluten-free Pizza

Week Two:

Meal	Monday	Tuesday	Wednesday	Thursday	Friday
Breakfast	Gluten-free French Toast	Rice Cereal with low FODMAP fruit	Lactose-free Yogurt with low FODMAP fruit	Blueberry Smoothie	Small Banana Pancakes
Lunch	Quinoa Bowl	Salad with Approved Dressing	Gluten-free Sandwich with Deli Meat and Cheese	Mixed Vegetable, Bean, and Pasta Soup	Tuna Salad on Gluten-free Bread
Dinner	Grilled Chicken with White Rice	Grilled Chicken Salad	Salad with Approved Dressing	Gluten-free Tacos	Stir-Fried Rice

Meal	Saturday	Sunday
Breakfast	Smoothie with low FODMAP fruit	Lactose-free Yogurt with low FODMAP fruit
Lunch	Rice Pasta with Marinara	Chicken Noodle Soup
Dinner	Baked Potato with Lactose-free Butter	Grilled Chicken Salad

Vegan 7-Day Meal Plan

Meal	Monday	Tuesday	Wednesday	Thursday	Friday
Breakfast	Coconut Yogurt with Chia Seeds	Rice Cakes with Peanut Butter	Corn Flakes with Almond Milk	Gluten-free Bread with Almond Butter	Unripe Banana with Coconut Yogurt
Lunch	Lemon and Garlic Roasted Zucchini	Rainbow Low FODMAP Slaw with Gluten-free Bread	Vegan Roasted Red Pepper Farfalle	Low FODMAP Coconut and Banana Cookie with Coconut Yogurt	Salad with Approved Dressing
Dinner	Low FODMAP Veggie Latkes	Gluten-free Pasta with Approved Sauce	Plain Tempeh with low FODMAP Veggie of choice	Plain Tofu with Rice Noodles	Gluten-free Pizza with Soy Cheese

Meal	Saturday	Sunday
Breakfast	Blueberry Smoothie with Coconut Milk	Banana and Oat Smoothie with Coconut Milk
Lunch	Plain Tofu with Soba Noodles	Plain Tempeh with Gluten-free Pasta
Dinner	Grilled Cabbage Soup	Baked Brussel Sprouts with Plain Tofu

Chapter 6: Low FODMAP diet tips and tricks for success

Starting a new diet can be scary. As we said before, your frame of mind is going to be incredibly important. It is vital you think about your why when making food choices. Each meal, we have a chance to better our health; all it takes is a little thought behind each decision.

Of course, we want to see you succeed with your diet. Below, you will find a number of tips and tricks that have helped other clients on the low FODMAP diet. While some may work for you, others may not. You must adjust the low FODMAP diet to match your desired lifestyle so you not only stick with it but can enjoy it at the same time!

1. Read the Label

Reading the labels on packaged foods is going to be vital for the success of your diet. Unfortunately, many high FODMAP ingredients can have very confusing names. We suggest carrying a list of additives to avoid until you learn them by heart. When you are more aware, you can avoid the high FODMAP ingredients.

2. Water-soluble

In general, low FODMAP foods are going to be water-soluble, but this does not mean they are fat-soluble. If you are cooking a soup with an onion, you will want to take the onion out. Instead, try using onion-infused oils for the taste. It is quick fix that may help with your IBS triggers.

1. High Fructose Corn Syrup

High Fructose Corn Syrup is in everything. Again, it will be important that you learn how to read food labels so you will be able to avoid this mistake. This ingredient is in a number of foods including energy bars, juices, mayonnaise, frozen meals, and even popcorn. Check the label before you put anything into your shopping cart.

2. Fiber

If you pick up a product and it seems to have a high serving f fiber, you can assume it is due to a high FODMAP additive. Try to avoid any products that boast about their fiber; it's a trap! Any fiber additives will more than likely trigger your GI issues.

3. Onion and Garlic Powder

When it comes to choosing out your spices, pay special attention to the labels. You will want to avoid onion and garlic powders as they contain high FODMAPs. Luckily, there are plenty of delicious low FODMAP approved spices as you can find in the chapter from above.

4. "Natural"

If you find any frozen foods, brothers, or savory soups that claim they have "natural" flavors, go ahead and check out the label. You can assume that they contain garlic and onion, very popular IBS triggers. You will want to try your best to avoid these additives to your meals.

5. "Healthy"

As much as we would like to trust when products claim they are healthy, this does not equate to low FODMAP approved. Foods like asparagus and apples are supposedly "healthy" for you, but they can trigger IBS symptoms. As you go through the elimination process, you will learn just what you can and cannot eat and make the decision if something is healthy for you.

6. Beverages

Often times, people forget that beverages can contain FODMAPs. You will want to pay special attention to what you are putting into your body. If you ever have questions, feel free to refer to our lists in the chapter from above. Just because a beverage claims it has no net carbohydrates, this does not mean they aren't high in FODMAPs.

7. Portion Control

While you are on the low FODMAP diet, portion is going to be key to success. When you are reading labels, you will always want to pay special attention to portion size. While a low FODMAP diet is approved, a bigger portion may still trigger IBS symptoms. You will want to try your best to be mindful of portion control.

8. Learn About Yourself

As you start this diet, you will want to spend plenty of time on the elimination phase. The more you test, the more you will be able to figure out what foods you can and cannot eat. When you have more to choose from, you will be able to get more creative with your recipes. At the end of the day, only you know what is best for you. When you learn yourself, the diet will become that much easier.

9. Food and Meal Journal

Your food and meal journal are going to be an important tool for your low FODMAP diet journey. By keeping track of the foods, you can and cannot eat; it will make it easier when you go back to check out your history. We eat so many different types of foods through the day; it can be hard to remember which foods trigger you. By keeping a journal, it leaves little room for mistakes.

10. Use Your Fridge

If you are trying your best to stick with the low FODMAP diet, why leave anything up to chance? Do yourself a favor and take the time to remove any high FODMAP foods in your house. By keeping your pantry and fridge stocked with the low FODMAP foods you need, it deletes any temptations you may have in the house.

11. Have A Backup Plan

Dieting is hard, especially when you are first starting out. When you are planning out your meals, it is possible to miss one here or there. Try to stack your freezer with low FODMAP meals so you can cook them in a few minutes. When your first plan falls through, you will always have a backup. It is a win-win situation!

Chapter 7: Low FODMAP diet FAQ

As we are nearing our time together, hopefully, you are feeling better about starting the low FODMAP diet. While you have learned a lot about the diet, feel free to check back whenever you have a question about the diet. Whether you need a refresher on the benefits of the diet or a reminder of which foods you can and cannot eat, you will be able to find the information here easily.

To finish off, we will hopefully be able to answer any further questions you have about the low FODMAP diet. Simply remember that this diet is going to be specifically tailored up to you. Being diagnosed with IBS or other GI tract issues is not the end of the world. It will take some extra effort, but when your symptoms and discomfort are relieved, you will be thankful you made the choice to start the low FODMAP diet. For now, it is time to answer some more popular questions you may still have.

Q. I am following the low FODMAP diet and still experiencing symptoms, is this the right diet for me?

A. The answer could be yes and no. If you are following the diet and still find yourself with symptoms of IBS, there may be another culprit in your diet. Remember to keep a food diet with you at all times so you can find any triggers you may be missing.

Q. Can I follow the low FODMAP diet as a vegetarian?

A. Absolutely! You can follow this diet whether you are vegan or vegetarian, it will just take a little extra work. You will find in the chapters before there are plenty of choices, so long as the allowed foods are not triggers for your own body. Some good sources of protein for this diet would be chickpeas, tofu, tempeh, and more. If there is a will, there is always a way!

Q. How do I make sure I'm getting enough Fiber?

A. This is one of the bigger concerns for those following the low FODMAP diet, especially if constipation is an issue. Luckily, several good low FODMAP sources can help you keep your fiber intake up. These include chia seeds, brown rice, flax seeds, kiwi, oranges, white potato, rice bran and more. Check out the list provided in the fourth chapter for a longer list.

Q. Should I eat Larger or Smaller Meals on the Low FODMAP Diet?

A. In general, you should try to eat three main meals through your day and to snacks between these meals. If you are still hungry, you can always add in another snack. Remember that portion control is going to be vital while you are on the low FODMAP diet, so this is something you will want to keep in mind when plating your meals.

Q. What is the rule with fats and oils on the Low FODMAP Diet?

A. As a general rule, there are plenty of fats and oils that are low in FODMAPs. However, anything in excess can trigger IBS symptoms. You will want to be especially aware of any condiments or sauces that are oil-based such as salad dressings. Most of the time, these also include high FODMAPs like garlic. Remember to always read the labels before consuming anything. You can also refer to our extended grocery list to see which fats and oils are allowed on the diet.

Q. Can I eat meat on the low FODMAP Diet?

A. Yes and No. Some sources of animal protein such as fish and chicken are low in FODMAPs. However, if the meat is prepared already, you will want to avoid any additives that may trigger your symptoms. If you have any further questions, please refer to the food lists from the chapter above.

Q. What happens if I break my diet?

A. While the aim of the diet is to stick to it as much as possible, mistakes and slip ups will happen. Overall, you will want to achieve control over any symptoms you may be having. If you slip up, expect to experience the IBS symptoms. As long as you return to your diet, you will most likely be able to improve them in a few days.

Q. Is this a lifestyle?

A. No, the low FODMAP diet is not meant to last for a lifetime. The aim of the diet is to help heal your gut over a controlled period of time. This diet should only be followed for two to six weeks. After this, you can begin to introduce food back into your diet. This will change depending on each individual.

PART II

For all the meat lovers out there, the next diet that we are going to discuss is known as the carnivore diet.

Chapter 1: What Is Carnivore Diet?

The Carnivore Diet is the all-new trendy diet that expects its followers to go on a meat-only way of lifestyle. This diet completely goes against nutritional stereotyping. If someone asked you to replace that bowl of meat with vegetable oils and carbs, you probably have been misled!

This diet has won favor for several reasons and is, of course, not a fluke. If you find it attractive to sink in a carnivore way of eating, you have come to the right place.

The carnivore diet is the one that entirely revolves around a meat-based pattern of eating. It is one extreme diet that restricts you from eating plant-based foods and strictly opposes carbohydrate consumption. It might sound crazy, but there are people including Shawn Baker (the creator of this diet) who have normalized this fact that carbohydrate is a non-essential macronutrient, and there is no harm in cutting them down from the menu.

It is a zero-carb diet that altogether emphasizes consuming meat. Scientists consider this diet the best nutrition source for human beings, cutting out the chatter from plant toxins.

There are more anecdotes and testimonials than research backed up with science. This no-carb diet has also been a second option to those who have either failed to carry on with Paleo and Keto diet or have faced other severe consequences after following them. This is a bold claim and has a lot to unpack. Let's dive deep into the depth of its science.

Researchers have carried out several studies throughout the Earth that has proved its benefits on humankind.

- **Removes the Inflammatory Vegetables -** If you have been suffering from an autoimmune disorder or a damaged gut, this might be of concern.

  Almost every vegetable has some kind of toxin in it. Brussels Sprouts, broccoli, cauliflower have sulforaphane that causes hypothyroidism and damage to health. Nightshades damage carb and fat metabolism. Polyphenols cause DNA damage. Lectins cause leaky guts. Reservatrol can inhibit androgen precursors. Spinach has oxalates that may result in kidney stones, and the list goes on. Choosing a carnivore diet can be a game-changing plan for such people and others who are still being manipulated by conventional nutritional advice.

- **It Increases Cholesterol –** You all must have heard about bad and good cholesterol. Cholesterol plays a negative role when it is oxidized or damaged and gets trapped in the artery walls. LDL cholesterol, even though it is given the tag of the 'bad' cholesterol, protects your body from diseases and does not cause them. They bind to the pathogens allowing the immune system to expel them.

During inflammation, the body uses LDL as a protective mechanism. So, people with heart diseases have high LDL levels because it binds to the pathogens, getting rid of the damage ensuring that it does not spread. It is, in fact, the inflammation that causes heart diseases.

- **It Increases the Nutrient Density** - Animal-based foods have the most bioavailable form of nutrients that play a crucial role from growth to brain function. While you have been a fiber-freak, you might just have missed out on the essential nutrients. Vegetarians have a deficiency in Vitamin B12 and Iron. Americans have Vitamin D deficiency, and women have Calcium deficiency, while Zinc is a deficient nutrient worldwide.

The brain requires micronutrients, and it is animals that mostly provide this. Zinc and iron are vital nutrients that help brain growth, dopamine transport, and serotonin synthesis.

- **It Reverses Insulin Resistance -** The best thing you could do to your health is reverse the insulin resistance. It is a problem where your body's cells become unresponsive to insulin action and therefore refuse to stuff the cells with more energy, leading to a rise in insulin level. It occurs due to excess carbohydrates and fat that shut off the process of burning fat, causing the fat to be stored without being used directly. The carnivore diet can be a solution to this!

- **Weight loss -** Since protein-based foods are satiating, they allow you to stay distracted from eating by making you feel fuller. By ingesting protein, the primary energy source is shifted from carbohydrate to fat. It is similar to ketosis (adapted to fat consumption), where you can use your body fat instead of carbohydrate.

Although it is as simple as a diet can be, the initial weeks can be hard. Here are the things that you can incorporate to get through the changeover conveniently:

- Before starting with the diet, you can get your blood test done since the metabolic needs vary with every individual.

- You might feel like giving up at some point, start getting headaches, and experience fatigue. It is normal as your body will be getting used to using energy from fat rather than carbohydrates.

- Your eating desire might fluctuate. You will get adjusted to this form of eating after one week.

Chapter 2: Recipes for Tasty Appetizers

If you are a meat lover and want to start the carnivore diet, here are some recipes for you to follow.

Oven-Baked Chicken Wings

Total Prep & Cooking Time: 1 hour 5 minutes

Yields: 8 servings

Nutrition Facts: Calories: 348 | Carbs: 1g | Protein: 25g | Fat: 27g | Fiber: 1g

Ingredients:

- Half cup of grated Parmesan
- Four pounds of chicken wings
- One tsp. of salt
- One tbsp. of parsley
- A quarter cup of grass-fed butter
- Half tsp. of black pepper (ground)

Method:

1. First of all, the oven needs to be preheated to 180 degrees Celsius or 350 degrees Fahrenheit.

2. Take a parchment paper for lining the baking sheet.

3. Now, you need to take a shallow bowl or dish for melting the butter.

4. In another clean bowl, mix parsley, pepper, Parmesan cheese, and salt.

5. Once the herb and cheese mixture is ready, dip the chicken wings in the bowl of melted butter one by one. After dipping, roll the wings in the mixture.

6. Arrange all the wings properly on top of the baking sheet.

7. Bake for an hour.

8. Take out the baked chicken wings from the oven and serve them warm.

Steak Nuggets

Total Prep & Cooking Time: 55-60 minutes

Yields: 4 servings

Nutrition Facts: Calories: 350 | Carbs: 1g | Protein: 40g | Fat: 20g | Fiber: 2g

Ingredients:

- One pound of beefsteak or venison steak (cut it into chunks)
- Palm or lard oil (needed for frying)
- One large-sized egg

For Keto Breading,

- Half cup each of
  - Pork panko
  - Parmesan cheese (grated)
- Half tsp. of seasoned salt (homemade)

For Chipotle Ranch Dip,

- A quarter cup each of
  - Organic cultured cream (sour)
  - Mayonnaise
- More than one tsp. of chipotle paste (for taste)
- A quarter medium-sized lime (juiced)

Method:

1. For preparing the Chipotle Ranch Dip, you need to combine all the ingredients and mix properly. Use either more or less chipotle paste in accordance to your taste preference. Refrigerate the dip before serving for a minimum of thirty minutes. You may store the dip for nearly a week.

2. Take a large-sized bowl and combine parmesan cheese, seasoned salt, and pork panko. Set aside after mixing evenly.

3. Now, beat one egg. Place the breading mix in one bowl and beaten egg in another.

4. Dip the steak chunks first in egg and then in the breading mix. Then, place them on a plate or sheet pan lined with wax paper.

5. Before frying, freeze the raw breaded steak bites for half an hour. By doing so, the breading won't lift at the time of frying.

6. Heat the lard to 325 degrees Fahrenheit. Fry the chilled or frozen steak nuggets for nearly two to three minutes until you get the brown color.

7. Keep the fried nuggets on a plate lined with a paper towel. Sprinkle a pinch of salt. Serve hot along with Chipotle Ranch.

Grilled Shrimp

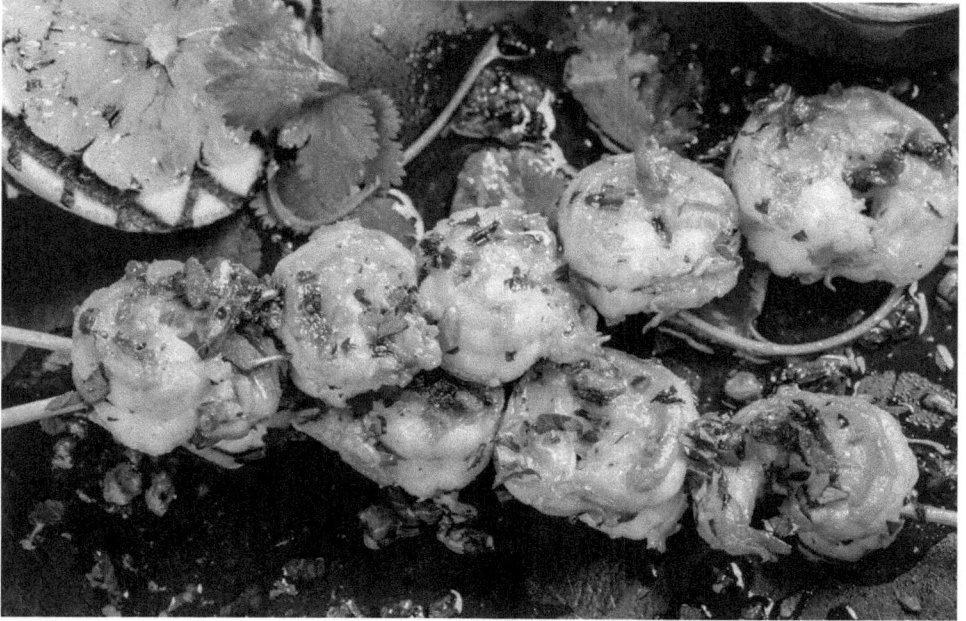

Total Prep & Cooking Time: 10 minutes

Yields: 4 servings

Nutrition Facts: Calories: 102 | Carbs: 1g | Protein: 28g | Fat: 3g | Fiber: 0g

Ingredients:

For grilling,

- One lb. of shrimp
- One tbsp. of lemon juice (freshly squeezed)

- Two tbsps. of olive oil (extra-virgin)
- For frying – vegetable oil or canola oil

For the shrimp seasoning,

- Half a tsp. of cayenne pepper
- One tsp. each of
  - Italian seasoning
  - Kosher salt
  - Garlic powder

Method:

1. You have to preheat your grill for this recipe on high.

2. Take a mixing bowl of large size, add all the ingredients of the seasoning in it and mix them well. Drizzle the lemon juice and olive oil into the mixture and keep stirring until you get a paste.

3. Add the shrimp into the bowl of seasonings and keep tossing so that all the pieces are evenly coated. Take the shrimp pieces and thread them onto wooden skewers.

4. Coat your grill with canola oil. You have to grill the shrimp for about three minutes for each side until they become opaque and pink.

5. Serve and enjoy!

Notes: You can store the grilled shrimp in the refrigerator for up to three days if you want to, but for the best flavor, you should consume it on the same day.

Roasted Bone Marrow

Total Prep & Cooking Time: 20 minutes

Yields: 2 servings

Nutrition Facts: Calories: 440 | Carbs: 0g | Protein: 4g | Fat: 48g | Fiber: 0g

Ingredients:

- To season – freshly ground black pepper and sea salt flakes
- Four bone marrow halves

Method:

1. Set the temperature of your oven to 350 degrees F and preheat.

2. Take a baking tray with deep sides and then place the bone marrow pieces in it.

3. Bake the bone marrow for half an hour until they become crispy and golden brown in color. The fat that is present in excess should have rendered off by now.

4. Season with black pepper and sea salt flakes.

5. You can spread the marrow separately on top of steaks, or you can serve the bone marrow as an appetizer.

Bacon-Wrapped Chicken Bites

Total Prep & Cooking Time: 30 minutes

Yields: 4 servings

Nutrition Facts: Calories: 230 | Carbs: 5g | Protein: 22g | Fat: 13g | Fiber: 1g

Ingredients:

- Three tbsps. of garlic powder
- Eight slices of thin bacon (slice them into one-third pieces)
- One chicken breast (large-sized, cut into bite-sized pieces)

Method:

1. Set the temperature of the oven to 400 degrees F and use aluminum foil to line the baking tray—Preheat the oven.

2. In a bowl, add the garlic powder. Take each chicken piece and dip it into the garlic powder.

3. Now, take each short piece of bacon and wrap it around the piece of chicken. Keep these prepared chicken pieces on the baking tray. Make sure they are not touching each other.

4. Bake the preparation for half an hour, and by the end of it, the bacon should turn crispy. After about fifteen minutes through pieces, turn the pieces over.

Salami Egg Muffins

Total Prep & Cooking Time: 25 minutes

Yields: 12 servings

Nutrition Facts: Calories: 142 | Carbs: 1g | Protein: 12g | Fat: 10g | Fiber: 0g

Ingredients:

- Four eggs (large-sized)
- Twenty slices of salami (uncured)
- Half a tsp. of kosher salt
- A quarter tsp. of black pepper
- Olive oil

Method:

1. Set the temperature of the oven to 350 degrees F and preheat. Take ramekins of four ounces each and spray them with olive oil. Then, place these ramekins on the baking sheet.

2. On the bottom of each ramekin, place one slice of salami and then on the sides, arrange four slices so that they are overlapping each other.

3. In this way, you will get a basket of salami, and in the middle of the basket, break one egg. Form four such baskets. Season the baskets with pepper and salt.

4. Bake the prepared salami baskets for twenty minutes, and by that time, they should be set.

5. Around the edges of the muffins, run a knife, and the muffins will get released. Serve and enjoy!

3-Ingredients Scotch Eggs

Total Prep & Cooking Time: 40 minutes

Yields: 12 servings

Nutrition Facts: Calories: 270 | Carbs: 1g | Protein: 19g | Fat: 20g | Fiber: 5g

Ingredients:

- Twelve large-sized boiled eggs
- Two pounds of chicken sausage or ground beef
- Two tsps. of salt

Method:

1. Preheating the oven to a temperature of 175 degrees Celsius or 350 degrees Fahrenheit is the first step for preparing such a delicious appetizer.

2. Line two baking sheets (small rimmed) with a parchment paper.

3. Take a large-sized bowl and combine chicken or beef and salt. Mix both the ingredients together by using your hands and then form twelve meatballs with it. Press the meatballs flat after placing them on top of the lined sheets.

4. Now, place each boiled egg inside each circle of flattened meat. After placing the eggs, start wrapping the meat nicely around the eggs. You are not supposed to leave any holes or gaps.

5. You need to bake for nearly fifteen minutes. Flip over as soon as the top looks cooked and again bake for ten minutes. If you want a crispy shell, then finish it under a broiler for approximately five minutes.

Notes: *If you are willing to enhance the taste, then you may feel free to add any of your favorite herbs, such as garlic or rosemary powder. Add one tsp. of your preferred herb into the meat just before wrapping the eggs. Hard-boiled eggs are better in this case as it is difficult to peel the soft boiled eggs.*

Chapter 3: Quick and Easy Everyday Recipes

Carnivore Waffles

Total Prep & Cooking Time: 6 minutes

Yields: 1 serving

Nutrition Facts: Calories: 274 | Carbs: 1g | Protein: 23.6g | Fat: 20.2g | Fiber: 0.8g

Ingredients:

- One-third cup of mozzarella cheese
- One egg
- Half cup of pork rinds (ground)
- A pinch of salt

Method:

1. For preparing the carnivore waffles, all you need is a waffle maker. First of all, preheat your waffle maker (medium-high heat).

2. Take a medium-sized bowl and whisk the pork rinds, cheese, and salt together.

3. Once you are done with the whisking part, pour the already prepared waffle mixture in the middle of the waffle maker's iron.

4. Close it and allow it to cook for three to five minutes. Or, you may cook until the waffle gets an attractive golden brown color.

5. Now, remove the cooked waffle and serve hot.

Notes: *The carnivore waffle will turn out to be more delicious if you place a cube of butter or runny egg on top of it. Greasing the waffle maker is not required before you start cooking waffles.*

Chicken Bacon Pancakes

Total Prep & Cooking Time: 20 minutes

Yields: 4 servings

Nutrition Facts: Calories: 444 | Carbs: 0g | Protein: 33g | Fat: 34g | Fiber: 0g

Ingredients:

- Four bacon slices
- Two chicken breasts
- Two tbsps. of coconut oil
- Four eggs (medium-sized, whisked)

Method:

1. First, you need to add all the ingredients to the bowl of the food processor except for the oil and then process everything together to form a smooth mixture.

2. After that, take your frying pan, and coconut oil to it.

3. From the batter that you just made, form four pancakes.

4. Fry these pancakes until they are set and properly cooked. Do the same with the rest of the batter.

Garlic Cilantro Salmon

Total Prep & Cooking Time: 25 minutes

Yields: 4 servings

Nutrition Facts: Calories: 294 | Carbs: 1g | Protein: 38.9g | Fat: 14.2g | Fiber: 0g

Ingredients:

- One lemon
- One fillet of salmon (large)
- A quarter cup of cilantro leaves (freshly chopped)
- Four garlic cloves (minced)
- One tablespoon of butter (optional)
- To taste – freshly ground black pepper and kosher salt

Method:

1. Set the temperature of the oven to 400 degrees F and preheat. Take a baking sheet and line it with foil. Place the fillets of salmon on it. You don't have to grease the foil.

2. Sprinkle the juice of one lemon over the fillet of salmon. Spread cilantro and garlic on top of the fillets evenly and season with pepper and salt. If

you want to use butter, then you have to place thin slices on top of the salmon fillet at this stage.

3. Now, place the salmon along with the foil in the oven and bake for about seven minutes.

4. Set broil settings and cook the salmon for an additional seven minutes. The top part should become crispy.

5. Use a flat spatula to remove the salmon from the oven. Separate the skin from the fish and serve!

Mustard-Seared Bacon Burgers

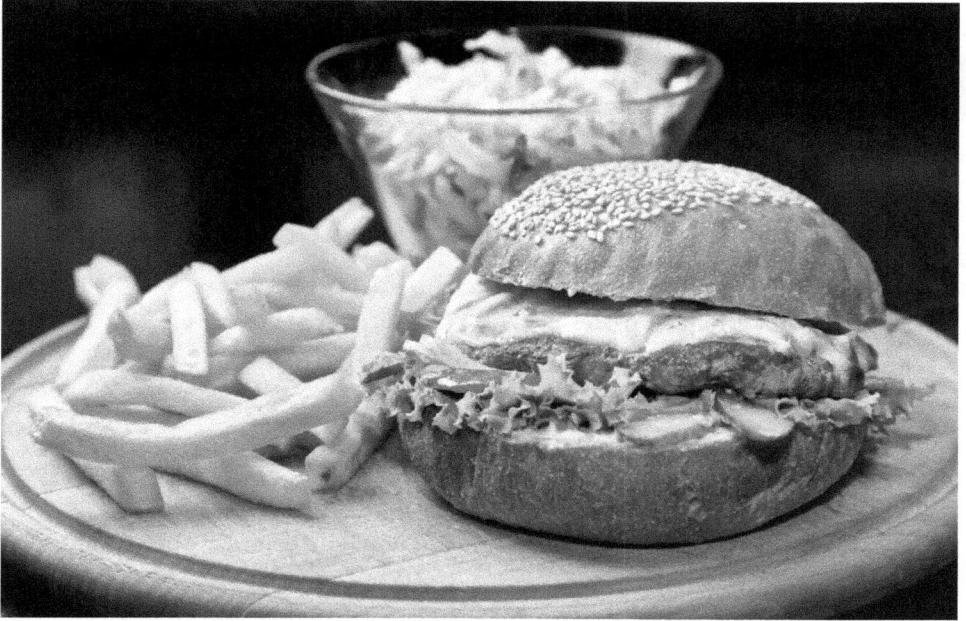

Total Prep & Cooking Time: 30 minutes

Yields: 6 servings

Nutrition Facts: Calories: 525 | Carbs: 3g | Protein: 22g | Fat: 45g | Fiber: 4g

Ingredients:

- 1.5 pounds of ground beef
- Four ounces of diced bacon
- Six tbsps. of yellow mustard
- To taste – salt and pepper

115

For the toppings,

- One tomato (properly diced)
- Half a red onion (diced)
- One avocado (thinly sliced)

For the sauce,

- Two tsps. of yellow mustard
- One tsp. of tomato paste
- A quarter cup of mayo

Method:

1. Take a pan and cook the bacon in it until it becomes crispy. You have to keep the grease of the bacon separately so that it can be used later. Then, take the bacon bits and keep them in a bowl along with the ground beef. Use pepper and salt to season them.

2. You will be able to form six patties from the mixture.

3. Now, you have to fry these burger patties on high flame so that they can get a great color. If you want, you can also choose to grill them.

4. Each patty will then have to be coated with one tbsp. of mustard and then, place the patty on the pan with the mustard-side facing down. Sear the patties one by one.

5. Take another bowl in which you can mix all the ingredients of the sauce together.

6. Each burger patty will have to be coated with sauce, and then, you can top them with slices of avocado, tomato, and onions.

Crockpot Shredded Chicken

Total Prep & Cooking Time: 6 hours

Yields: 8 servings

Nutrition Facts: Calories: 201 | Carbs: 1g | Protein: 24g | Fat: 10g | Fiber: 0g

Ingredients:

- Four garlic cloves
- Four chicken breasts
- One cup of chicken broth
- Half an onion (sliced)
- One tbsp. of Italian seasoning
- To taste – Salt and pepper

Method:

1. Take all the ingredients and add them to the crockpot.

2. Cook them for about six hours on low.

3. Use forks to shred the meat.

4. You can enjoy the shredded chicken with a variety of dishes like sautés, lettuce wraps, salads, or even soups.

Chapter 4: Weekend Dinner Recipes

Organ Meat Pie

Total Prep & Cooking Time: 20 minutes

Yields: 4 servings

Nutrition Facts: Calories: 412 | Carbs: 2g | Protein: 35g | Fat: 28g | Fiber: 4.2g

Ingredients:

- Half pound each of
  - Beef liver (ground)
  - Beef heart (ground)
  - Ground beef
- Three eggs
- Butter, ghee or Homemade Tallow or any melted cooking fat
- Salt (as required)

Method:

1. The oven needs to be preheated to 175 degrees Celsius or 350 degrees Fahrenheit.

2. Take a mixing bowl: mix ground beef, beef heart, and beef liver along with eggs and cooking fat of your choice. Lastly, add salt into the mixture.

3. Now, take a pie plate of nine inches and grease it lightly. Pour the mixture into the pie plate evenly.

4. Bake it for nearly fifteen to twenty minutes. Or, you may bake until the egg is totally set.

5. After baking, remove the pie from direct heat and let it cool for about five minutes. Serve it in a warm condition. In the case of leftovers, enjoy it cold.

Notes: *For those of you who are willing to add flavor to this recipe, you may add half tbsp. of any seasoning mix with the meat.*

Smokey Bacon Meatballs

Total Prep & Cooking Time: 30 minutes

Yields: 8 servings

Nutrition Facts: Calories: 280 | Carbs: 1g | Protein: 13g | Fat: 25g | Fiber: 0g

Ingredients:

- Two garlic cloves (skins peeled)
- Eight bacon slices (crumbled and cooked)
- One pound ground chicken or two chicken breasts
- One egg (properly whisked)
- Two drops of liquid smoke
- One tbsp. of onion powder
- Four tbsps. of olive oil

Method:

1. First, take all the ingredients (except for the oil) and add them to the bowl of the food processor and mix everything.

2. You will be able to form about twenty to twenty-four meatballs from the mixture. These balls will be small in size.

3. Now, take a large-sized frying pan, and then heat the oil. Add the meatballs and fry them until they are browned. It will take about five minutes for each side. If you want them to be perfect, then avoid overcrowding and cook in batches.

Steak au Poivre

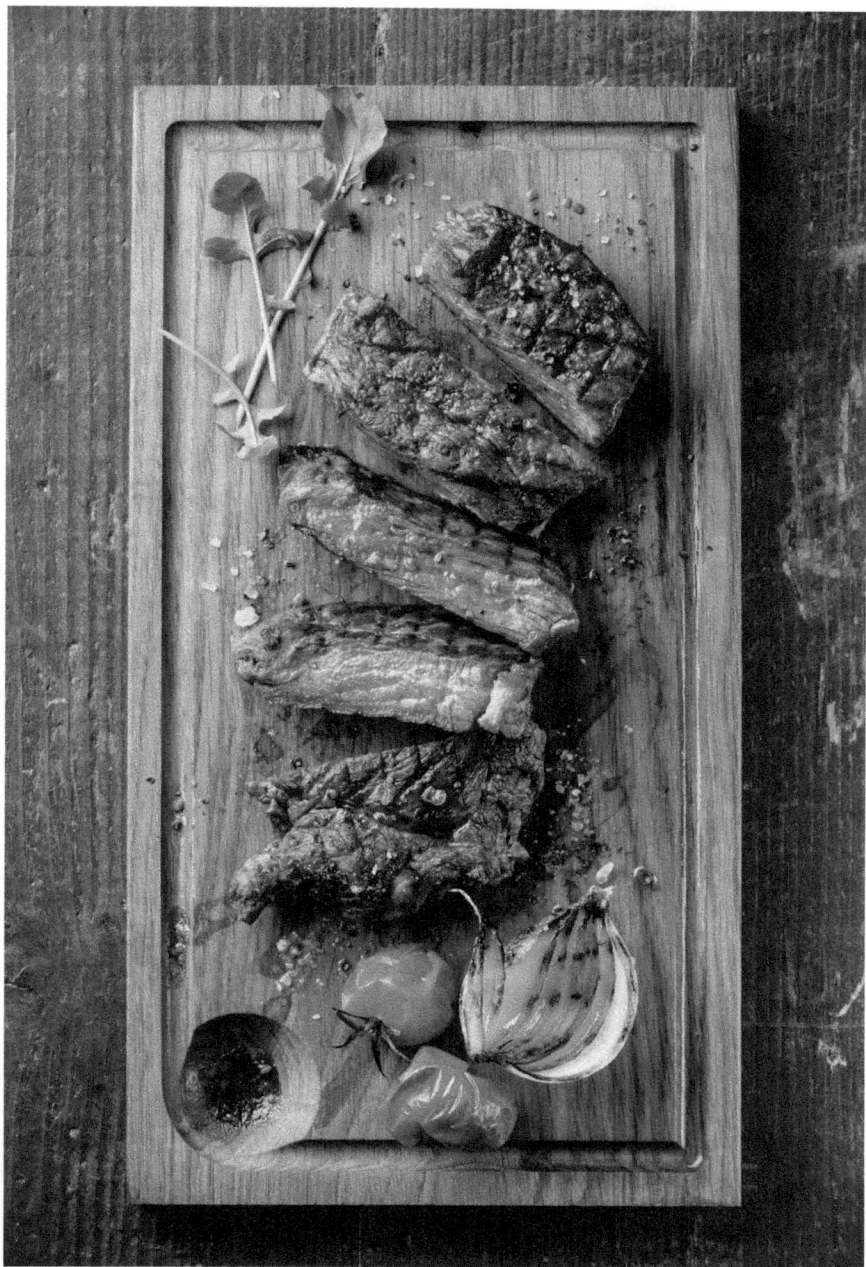

Total Prep & Cooking Time: 15 minutes

Yields: 1 serving

Nutrition Facts: Calories: 696 | Carbs: 2g | Protein: 42g | Fat: 58g | Fiber: 0g

Ingredients:

- One fillet of mignon (approximately six ounces)
- One thyme sprig
- One tbsp. of salt
- Two tbsps. each of
  o Ghee
  o Peppercorns
- Two garlic cloves (minced)

Method:

1. After you take the steaks out of the refrigerator, season them nicely with salt and then allow them to sit for about half an hour.

2. Use a mortar and pestle to crush the peppercorns completely on a pan or a flat board.

3. Take the steak, and on both sides of it, press the crushed peppercorns.

4. Place a skillet on the oven and heat it. Add the ghee. After that, sauté the thyme and garlic.

5. When you notice that the ghee has become hot, place the pieces of steak in the pan. Cook each side for about four minutes. The end result will be medium-rare steak.

Skillet Rib Eye Steaks

Total Prep & Cooking Time: 55 minutes

Yields: 2 servings

Nutrition Facts: Calories: 347 | Carbs: 1g | Protein: 22g | Fat: 14.2g | Fiber: 0g

Ingredients:

- Two tsps. of freshly chopped rosemary leaves
- One tsp. of seasoning of your choice
- One tbsp. each of
  - Olive oil
  - Unsalted butter
- One rib-eye steak (bone-in)

Method:

1. Take the sheet pan and on it, place the rib-eye steak. Use the seasoning to coat both sides properly. Spread the rosemary leaves on top.

2. Now, keep this steak in the refrigerator for three days after covering. Before cooking, take the steak out and keep it outside at room temperature for half an hour.

3. Place a skillet on the oven and heat it. Add olive oil and butter and wait until all of the butter has melted. Coat the skillet properly with butter by tilting the pan.

4. Now, add the steak to the skillet and cook for about five minutes until you notice that the bottom side has become caramelized and browned. After that, flip it over and baste the other side with oil and butter and cook it for five more minutes.

5. Take the steak off from the pan and slice it into thin pieces after it has cooled down for about five minutes.

Pan-Fried Pork Tenderloin

Total Prep & Cooking Time: 20 minutes

Yields: 2 servings

Nutrition Facts: Calories: 330 | Carbs: 0g | Protein: 47g | Fat: 15g | Fiber: 0g

Ingredients:

- One tbsp. of coconut oil
- To taste – pepper and salt
- One pound of pork tenderloin

Method:

1. Start by cutting the pork tenderloin in two halves.

2. Place your frying pan on the oven on medium flame. Add the oil in the pan and heat it.

3. Once the oil has melted completely, place the two pieces of the pork tenderloin in the oil.

4. Allow the pieces to cook thoroughly. Use tongs to flip the pieces so that all the sides of the pork are evenly cooked.

5. Take a reading on the thermometer, and it should show that the temperature is just below 63 degrees C or 145 degrees F.

6. Allow the pork to cool down after you take it out and then use a sharp knife to cut it into small pieces.

Carnivore Chicken Enchiladas

Total Prep & Cooking Time: 30 minutes

Yields: 10 servings

Nutrition Facts: Calories: 271 | Carbs: 5g | Protein: 25g | Fat: 7g | Fiber: 1.5g

Ingredients:

- Two chicken breasts (skinless, boneless)
- Three tbsps. of bottles lime juice + juice of one fresh lime
- One tsp. of dried garlic
- 16 oz. of sliced chicken
- Chimichurri sauce
- One jar of enchilada sauce
- One bell pepper (thinly sliced)
- Eight oz. each of
  - Cooked spinach
  - Shredded cheese

Method:

For making the shredded chicken,

1. First, take a crockpot and add the shredded pieces of chicken in it. Add the lime juice too.

2. Sprinkle the Chimichurri sauce on top of the chicken and then sprinkle the garlic on top.

3. Now, cook the chicken for about 4-5 hours if you want to cook it on high. Alternatively, if you're going to cook it on low, then set it for 8 hours.

4. Once it is done, use a fork to shred the chicken.

Assembling the enchiladas,

1. Set the temperature of your oven to 400 degrees F and preheat.

2. Take all the other ingredients like pepper and spinach and prep them.

3. The enchilada wrapped will be made by the four slices of chicken.

4. In the middle of the wrapper, add the shredded chicken.

5. Then, on either side, add the cooked spinach, pepper, and some of the cheese.

6. Roll the wrappers carefully and make sure they are firm.

7. Once you have rolled them completely, place them in a pan with the seam sides facing downwards. Then, add the enchilada sauce all over them.

8. Take the remaining portion of the cheese and sprinkle on top of the enchiladas. Bake the preparation for about fifteen minutes in the oven.

9. Serve and enjoy!

•

PART III

Be gentle with yourself throughout this process as it will be uncomfortable at times and will require strength. This book will help you through it, as you are not alone. I hope that this book also reminds you that many other people are suffering from the same type of food-related disorders as you are and that you are not alone in that either. This book will take a step-by-step approach, which will make for the highest chance of recovery. If at any time you need to take a break in order to think about the information you have learned, feel free to do so, but make sure you come back to this book quite soon after. Going through this process of recovery can be a lot, but with the right support, it will be possible.

You have already taken the first step in recovery, which is acknowledging that you have an issue. For that, I congratulate you!

What Is Emotional Eating?

Emotional eating occurs when a person suffering from emotional deficiencies of some sort, including lack of affection, lack of connection, or other factors like stress, depression, anxiety, or even general negative feelings like sadness or anger, eats in order to gain comfort from the food they are eating.

Many people find comfort in food. When people experience negative feelings and turn to food consumption in order to reduce their pain or to feel better, this is called emotional eating.

Now, some people do this on occasion like after a breakup or after a bad fight, but when this occurs at least a few times a week, this is when it is considered to have a negative impact on one's life and is when it becomes an issue that needs to be addressed.

What Is Binge Eating?

Binge eating disorder is another disorder that can be seen along with emotional eating. Binge eating disorder is when a person eats much more than a regular amount of food in a single occasion or sitting, and they feel unable to control themselves or to stop themselves. This could also be defined as a compulsion to overeat. In order to be considered a disorder, it has to happen at least two times per week for longer than six months consecutively.

Along with binge eating is overeating, although this is also sometimes seen as a separate disorder altogether. Overeating is when a person eats more than they require in order to sustain life. This occurs when they consume much more than they need in a day, or in a single sitting.

Overeating does not necessarily become binge eating, but it certainly can. Overeating is a general term used to describe the eating disorders that we just defined-Emotional Eating and Binge Eating. Thus, overeating could involve binge eating, food addiction, or other food-related disorders.

In this book, we will be focusing on emotional eating and binge eating, and how you can overcome these two food-related disorders.

What Is Bulimia?

Bulimia is another eating disorder. Bulimia involves binge eating, followed by extreme feelings of shame, guilt, and disdain for oneself and one's body. This is accompanied by intense feelings of body dysmorphia and body image issues, as well as the desire to be "skinnier." Thus, the person will turn to purging- or self-inflicted vomiting in an effort to lose weight and rid themselves of the guilt and shame.

Chapter 1: Understanding Your Food-Related Disorder

In this chapter, we are going to look at these two food-related disorders (binge eating/ bulimia and emotional eating) in much more detail. We will begin by looking at the most common reasons why people suffer from these disorders and will spend some time examining scientific research about why these disorders exist.

Why Do People Eat Emotionally?

The reason that emotional eating occurs is that eating foods that we enjoy makes us feel rewarded on an emotional and physiological level within our brain.

Why Do People Binge Eat?

People binge eat for a very similar reason to the reason why people experience emotional eating. This is because eating foods that we enjoy in terms of taste, smell, texture, and so on, makes us feel rewarded on an emotional and physiological level within our brains.

Throughout the rest of this chapter, we will look more in-depth at these eating disorders in order to give you more information about why they occur and what could cause them.

Scientific Research on Eating Disorders and Why They Exist

You may be asking how food cravings can result from emotional deficiencies and how these two seemingly unrelated things can be considered related. While we have touched on this briefly in this book already, the reason for this is that your body learns, over time, that eating certain foods makes it feel rewarding, positive, and happy for some time after it is ingested. These foods include convenience foods such as those containing processed sugars or salts, fast food, and quick pastries.

When you are sad or worried, your body feels negative and looks for ways to remedy this. Your brain then connects these two facts- that the body does not feel positive and that it wants to find a way to fix this. The brain then decides that eating the foods that make it feel good will remedy the situation. This process happens in the background of your mind without you being aware of it, and it leads you to consciously feel a craving for those specific foods such as sugary snacks or salty fast-food meals. You may not even be aware of why. If you then decide to give in to this craving and eat something like a microwave pizza snack, your body will feel rewarded and happy for a brief period of time. This reinforces to your brain that turning to food in an effort to make yourself feel better emotionally has been successful.

If you end up feeling down and guilty that you ate something that was unhealthy or that you ate too much, your brain will again try and remedy these negative emotions by craving food. This is how a cycle of emotional eating or a cycle of bingeing and purging can begin and continue. This could happen largely in your subconscious without you being any the wiser.

Why Do People Have Bulimia or Other Food Disorders?

Because scientists and psychiatrists understand this process that occurs in the brain, they know that food cravings can indicate emotional deficiencies. While there are other types of cravings that can occur, such as those that pregnant ladies experience, or those that indicate nutrient deficiencies, there are ways to tell that a craving is caused by some type of emotional deficiency.

It begins by determining the foods that a person craves and when they crave them. If every time someone has a stressful situation, they feel like eating a pizza, or if a person who is depressed tends to eat a lot of chocolate, this could indicate emotional eating. As you know by now, emotional eating and bulimia are closely related, and emotional eating can lead to bulimia over time.

If you crave fruit like a watermelon on a hot day, you are likely just dehydrated, and your body is trying to get water from a water-filled fruit that it knows will make it more hydrated. Examining situations like this has led scientists and psychiatrists to explore eating disorders in more depth and determine what types of emotional deficiencies can manifest themselves through food cravings or disordered eating in this way.

In the next chapter, we will look at psychological triggers that can lead to disordered eating.

The Neuroscience of Brain Chemicals and Food As a Reward

Many times, we may see ingredients on the packages of foods we eat, but we aren't really sure of exactly what they are, just that they taste good. In this section, we will take a deeper look at them and what they do to your brain.

Casein is a heavily processed ingredient that is derived from milk. It is processed a few times over and eventually creates milk solids that are concentrated. These milk solids- called Casein are then added into foods like cheese, french fries, milkshakes, and other fast and convenient packaged or fast-foods that contain dairy or dairy products (such as pastries and salad dressings). Casein has been compared to nicotine in its addictive properties. It is often seen in cheese, and this is why there is increasing evidence that people can become, and many are already addicted to cheese. The reason for this is during digestion. When cheese and other foods that contain casein are digested, it is broken down, and one of the compounds that it breaks down into is a compound that is strikingly similar to opioids- the highly addictive substance that is in pain killers.

High fructose corn syrup is surely an ingredient you have heard of before or at least one that you have seen on the packaging of your favorite snacks or quick foods. While this is actually derived from real corn, after it is finished being processed, there is nothing corn-like about it. High fructose corn syrup is essentially the same thing as refined sugar when all is said and done. It is used as a sweetener in foods like soda, cereal, and other sweet and quick foods. The reason why this ingredient is seen so often is that it is much cheaper than using sugar and is much easier to work with. High Fructose Corn Syrup is another common food additive that has been shown to be highly addictive. This substance has been shown to be similar to cocaine in its addictive properties.

MSG stands for Monosodium Glutamate, which sounds a lot like a chemical you may have encountered in science class in college. MSG is added to foods to give it a delicious flavor. It is essentially a very concentrated form of salt. What this does in foods such as fast-food, packaged convenience foods, and buffet-style food is that it gives it that wonderfully salty and fatty flavor that makes us keep coming back for more. Companies put this in food because it comes at an extremely low cost, and the flavor it brings covers up the artificial flavors of all of the other cheap ingredients that are used to make these foods. MSG has been known to block our natural appetite suppressant, which normally kicks in when we have had enough to eat. For this reason, when we are eating foods containing MSG, we do not recognize when we are satiated, and we continue to eat until we are stuffed because it tastes so great.

Chapter 2: Understanding Your Mind

In this chapter, we are going to look at some of the psychological factors that can lead to disordered eating so that you can gain a better understanding of what could have led you to use food as a means of coping.

Psychological and Emotional Triggers

There are several types of emotional deficiencies that can be indicated by disordered eating. We will explore these in detail below in hopes that you will recognize some of the reasons why you may be struggling with an eating disorder.

Childhood Causes

The first example of an emotional deficiency that we will examine is more of an umbrella for various emotional deficiencies. This umbrella term is Childhood Causes. If you think back on your childhood, think about how your relationship with food was cultivated. Maybe you were taught that when you behaved, you received food as a reward. Maybe when you were feeling down, you were given food to cheer you up. Maybe you turned to food when you were experiencing negative things in your childhood. Any of these could cause someone to suffer from emotional eating in their adulthood, as it had become something learned. This type is quite difficult to break as it has likely been a habit for many, many years, but it is possible. When we are children, we learn habits and make associations without knowing it that we often carry into our later lives. While this is no fault of yours, recognizing it as a potential issue is important to make changes.

Covering Up Emotions

Another emotional deficiency that can manifest itself in emotional eating and food cravings is actually the effort to cover up our emotions. Sometimes we would rather distract ourselves and cover up our emotions than to feel them or to face them head-on. In this case, our brain may make us feel hungry in an effort to distract us from the act of eating food. When we have a quiet minute where these feelings or thoughts would pop into our minds, we can cover them up by deciding to prepare food and eat and convince ourselves that we are "too busy" to acknowledge our feelings because we have to deal with our hunger. The fact that it is hunger that arises in this scenario makes it very difficult to ignore and very easy to deem as a necessary distraction since, after all, we do need to eat in order to survive. This can be a problem though, if we are not in need of nourishment, and we are telling ourselves that this is the reason why we cannot deal with our demons or our emotions. If there is something that you think you may be avoiding dealing with or thinking about or if you tend to be very uncomfortable with feelings of unrest, you may be experiencing this type of emotional eating.

Feeling Empty or Bored

When we feel bored, we often decide to eat or decide that we are hungry. This occupies our mind and our time and makes us feel less bored and even feel positive and happy. We also may eat when we are feeling empty. When we feel empty the food will quite literally be ingested in an effort to fill a void, but as we know, the food will not fill a void that is emotional in sort, and this will lead to an unhealthy cycle of trying to fill ourselves emotionally with something that will never actually work. This will lead us to become disappointed every time and continue trying to fill this void with material things like food or purchases. This can also be a general feeling of dissatisfaction with life and feelings of lacking something in your life. Looking deeper into this the next time you feel those cravings will be difficult but will help you greatly in the long term as you will then be able to identify the source of your feelings of emptiness and begin to fill these voids in ways that will be much more effective.

Affection Deficiency

Another emotional deficiency that could manifest itself as food cravings is an affection deficiency. This type of deficiency can be feelings of loneliness, feelings of a lack of love, or feelings of being undesired. If a person has been without an intimate relationship or has recently gone through a breakup, or if a person has not experienced physical intimacy in quite some time, they may be experiencing an affection deficiency. This type of emotional deficiency will often manifest itself in food cravings as we will try to gain feelings of comfort and positivity from the good tasting, drug-like (as we talked about in chapter one) foods they crave.

Low Self-Esteem

Another emotional deficiency that may be indicated by food cravings is a low level of self-esteem. Low self-esteem can cause people to feel down, unlovable, inadequate, and overall negative and sad. This can make a person feel like eating foods they enjoy will make them feel better, even if only for a few moments. Low self-esteem is an emotional deficiency that is difficult to deal with as it affects every area of a person's life, such as their love life, their social life, their career life, and so on. Sometimes people have reported feeling like food was something that was always there for them, and that never left them. While this is true, they will often be left feeling even emptier and lower about themselves after giving into cravings.

Mood

A general low mood can cause emotional eating. While the problem of emotional eating is something that is occurring multiple times per week and we all have general low moods or bad days, if this makes you crave food and especially food of an unhealthy sort, this could become emotional eating. If every time we feel down or are having a bad day, we want to eat food to make ourselves feel better; this is emotional eating. Some people will have a bad day and want a drink at the end of the day, and if this happens every once in a while, it is not necessarily a problem with emotional eating. The more often it happens, the more often it is emotional eating. Further, we do not have to give in to the cravings for it to be considered emotional eating. Experiencing the cravings often and in tandem with negative feelings in the first place is what constitutes emotional eating.

Depression

Suffering from depression also can lead to emotional eating. Depression is a constant low mood for a period of months on end, and this low mood can cause a person to turn to food for comfort and a lift in spirit. This can then become emotional eating in addition to and because of depression.

Anxiety

Having anxiety can lead to emotional eating, as well. There are several types of anxiety, and whether it is general anxiety (constant levels of anxiety), situational anxiety (triggered by a situation or scenario), it can lead to emotional eating. You have likely heard of the term *comfort food* to describe certain foods and dishes. The reason for this is because they are usually foods rich in carbohydrates, fats, and heavy in nature. These foods bring people a sense of comfort. These foods are often turned to when people suffering from anxiety are emotionally eating because these foods help to temporarily ease their anxiety and make them feel calmer and more at ease. This only lasts for a short period of time; however, before their anxiety usually gears up again.

Stress

Stress eating is probably the most common form of emotional eating. While this does not become an issue for everyone experiencing stress, and many people will do so every once in a while, it is a problem for those who consistently turn to food to ease their stress. Some people are always under stress, and they will constantly be looking for ways to ease their stress. Food is one of these ways that people use to make themselves feel better and to take their minds off of their stress. As with all of the other examples we have seen above, this is not a lasting resolution, and it becomes a cycle. Similar to the cycle diagram we saw above, the same can be used for stress except instead of a negative emotion and eating making you feel more down, stress eating can make you feel more stress as you feel like you have done something you shouldn't have which causes you stress, and the cycle ensues.

Recognizing your triggers is important because this will allow you to notice when you may be feeling emotional hunger and when you are feeling actual hunger. If you become hungry, you can look back on your day or on the last hour and determine if any of your triggers were present. If they were, then you will be able to determine that you are likely experiencing emotional hunger, and you can take the appropriate steps instead of giving in to the cravings blindly.

There are many different emotional causes for the cravings we experience. There may be others than those listed above, and these are all valid. A person's emotional eating experience is unique and personal and could be caused by any number of things. You may also experience a combination of emotional deficiencies listed above, or one of those listed above in addition to others. Many of these can overlap, such as anxiety and depression, which are often seen together in a single person. The level of these emotional deficiencies that you experience could indicate the level of emotional eating that you struggle with. Whatever your experience and your struggles though, there is hope of recovery, and this is what the rest of this book will focus on.

Chapter 3: How to Stop Binge Eating, Bulimia, and Emotional Eating

In this chapter, we are going to look at how you can begin to tackle your mind in order to make positive changes for your body and break free from your eating disorder once and for all.

Addressing the Core Wounds

The key to solving these food-related issues is to address your core wounds. Understanding how your mind works will help you to better take care of it. You will be able to recognize your feelings and how they could have come about, and then treat them in a way that will help it to feel better. Bettering your relationship with food and your body will also improve your relationship with your mind. This will then allow you to begin to feed it what it needs, which will, in turn, lead to better cognitive functioning, control over impulses, and decision-making. This will help overall in your relationship with your food, your body, and your mind.

What Are Core Wounds?

As we discussed in the previous chapter, there are several types of emotional deficiencies that can be indicated by disordered eating. Once you have determined which of these emotional deficiencies (or which combination of them) are present in your life, you can begin to look at them in a little more detail. By doing so, you will come upon your core wounds. A core wound is something that you believe to be true about yourself or your life, and it is something that likely came about as a result of a coping mechanism you developed to deal with childhood. For example, this could be something like; the feeling of not being enough, the belief that you are unlovable, or the belief that you are stupid.

How to Address Them

By understanding and addressing your core wounds, you will be able to change your behaviors because of the intricate relationship that exists between your thoughts, your emotions, and your behaviors. By addressing your thoughts and emotions, you will change your behaviors and thus, free yourself from disordered eating. You may be wondering how you can begin to address your core wounds, as it can be difficult to know where to begin.

The first step is learning how to control and change your thoughts, which in turn, leads to changes in your behavior. By taking control of your thoughts and your beliefs, they don't have the opportunity to manifest into unhealthy behaviors such as overeating, turning to food for comfort, or any other unhealthy coping mechanisms that you have developed over the course of your life.

Becoming aware of your own thoughts is the most crucial step in this entire guide, as everything else will fail without it. Paying attention to your thoughts will help you identify what thoughts are going through your mind during an intense emotional moment. By looking deep within, in order to get in touch with your deepest feelings, you will be more likely to succeed in your weight loss and your overall lifestyle improvement.

One great example of how to put this into practice is through the use of journaling. Journaling can help in a process such as this because it can help you to organize your thoughts and feelings and will help you to see visually what is working and what isn't working for you. While we can give tips and examples, every person is different, so to find exactly what works for you, you will have to try some different things and see which techniques help you personally the most and in the best way. Journaling can be about anything like how you feel since beginning a new program, how you feel physically since changing your diet, how you feel emotionally now that you are not reaching for food in order to comfort your emotions and anything along the lines of this.

Positive Self-Talk

Once you have addressed your emotions and your core wounds, you can begin to intervene and change them so that they result in healthier behaviors. You will do this using positive self-talk. Adopting helpful thought processes fosters better emotions overall, which leads to more productive behaviors.

When people have developed unhelpful thinking processes, it is hard to make decisions to benefit their future selves because their thoughts create negative emotions that drive away motivation. This is where something called *positive self-talk* can come in. Positive self-talk can be instrumental in helping you to recover from disordered eating.

What Is Positive Self-Talk?

Many people's minds are controlled by their inner critic. The inner critic shares words with you, such as "You should just give up" Or "What makes you think you'll succeed?" which is rooted in the opposite of positive self-talk- Negative self-talk!

Instead of creating an open space that allows for mistakes, growth, and development, your inner critic causes you to question your worth, which makes it difficult for you to have the positive, growth mindset that is needed to complete tasks and go after things that may be difficult to achieve. In this case, helping your mind to begin using positive self-talk will help you to recover for the long-term.

How to Use Positive Self-Talk?

Below are several ways that you can begin to use positive self-talk. Over time, your mind will get used to thinking in this way, and you will find it much easier to do.

1. Remind yourself

Bad habits are built through many years, and no amount of willpower can undo a lifetime of bad habits, such as a strong inner critic that uses negative self-talk. By rewiring your brain to minimize the amount of negativity you feel in the first place, you will eventually get used to filling your mind with positive thoughts instead of negative ones.

2. Stop the automatic process of negativity

Often times, if the person had just paid attention to their thought process, they would be able to catch themselves before their mind automatically spiraled to a place of complete de-motivation. By catching yourself before you get there, you can prevent yourself from falling into your negative thought patterns that are limiting you and holding you back.

3. Find positive influences

Surrounding yourself with people that can encourage you and foster positivity will also change your inner-critic's opinion. Often times, hearing positive compliments from other people hold a heavier weight in the eyes of your inner-critic compared to you telling your inner-critic the same thing. Try spending time with people who are supportive of your goals and the changes that you are looking to make in your life. It will make your journey a little bit easier.

4. Limit Negative Influences

By limiting the negative influences in your life, you are making a statement to yourself that you place importance on preserving your mental health. When you remove negative influences and limit your exposure to things or people that make you feel negative, you are prioritizing yourself, and this is a great way to practice self-care.

5. Practice a gratitude exercise

This is a great exercise to remind yourself of everything that you love and appreciate about yourself and your life. Take time to write down all of the things that you love about yourself and about your life. This will remind you of all of the positivity surrounding you and will serve to uplift you.

Chapter 4: Making Healthier Decisions Using Intuitive

Eating

This chapter will provide you with a solid foundation of knowledge on which to build your new lifestyle. We will look at how intuitive eating can be the answer to all of your struggles and help you to find recovery.

Making Good Choices

As we discussed in the previous chapter, making good choices begins with self-exploration and a deep look into your core wounds. Once you have done this, you can begin to make decisions that are positive for your health and your life, and over time these will become more and more habitual. We are going to spend this chapter looking at some of the ways that you can begin to make good choices related to food and eating.

How to Begin Making Good Choices Using Intuitive Eating

One great way to make good choices when it comes to food is by using something called intuitive eating. Below, I will define intuitive eating for you and give you some insight into how this can change your life.

What Is Intuitive Eating?

Intuitive eating is a new perspective from which to view how you feed your body. This style of eating puts you in control, instead of following a list of pre-designed guidelines about when and what to eat. Intuitive eating instead encourages you to listen to your body and the signals it sends you about what, how much, and when to eat. This ensures that you are giving your body exactly what it needs when it needs it, instead of forcing it into a specific kind of diet.

Intuitive eating does not limit any specific foods and does not require you to stick to certain foods exclusively. Instead, it encourages you to learn as much as you can about what your body is telling you and follow its signals.

The two main components of the intuitive eating philosophy are the following; eat when you are hungry and stop eating when you are satiated. This may seem like a no-brainer, but in today's societies, we are very far from eating in an intuitive way, as odd as it may seem. With so many diet trends and numerous "rules" for how you should and should not eat, it can be difficult to put these ideas aside and let your body guide you exclusively.

Intuitive Eating and Hunger

Before we begin looking at the specifics of intuitive eating, we will look at the different types of hunger and how you can tell them apart. This will help you to distinguish when you are hungry and when you may be turning to food to soothe your emotional state.

Real hunger is when our body needs nutrients or energy and is letting us know that we should replenish our energy soon. This happens when it has been a few hours since our last meal when we wake up in the morning, or after a lot of strenuous activity like a long hike. Our body uses hunger to signal to us that it is in need of more energy and that if it doesn't get it soon, it will begin to use our stored energy as fuel. While there is nothing wrong with our body using its stored fuel, it can be used as a sign to us that we should eat shortly in order to replenish these stores. Perceived Hunger is when we think we are hungry, but our body doesn't actually require any more energy or for the stores to be replenished. This can happen for a number of reasons, including an emotional deficiency, a negative mental state, or the occurrence of a psychological trigger.

The philosophy behind intuitive eating is that if you wait until you are too hungry before eating, you will be much more likely to overeat or to binge eat. This is because, by this time, you be feeling ravenous instead of mildly hungry. If instead, you choose to adhere to your hunger and eat when your body tells you that it needs sustenance, you will be much more likely to eat just the right amount. As a result, your body will be satisfied rather than completely stuffed, and instead of feeling shameful and angry that you have eaten, you can feel happy that you have provided your body with what it needed. This requires you to listen to and respect what your body is telling you and then provide it with nutrients in order for it to keep working hard for you!

The Benefits of Intuitive Eating

One of the reasons that intuitive eating is such a successful and cherished form of eating is that it allows the body to lead the mind in the right direction when it comes to seeking out its needs. Below, we will look at the benefits of letting your body guide your eating choices.

- Allows the body to get what it needs

Did you know that your cravings could actually be giving you much more information than you give them credit for?
A craving is an intense longing for something (in this case food), that comes about intensely and feels urgent. In our case, that longing is for s a very specific type of food. When we have cravings for certain foods, it can actually mean more than what it seems.

While you may think that a craving is an indication of hunger or of a desire for the taste of a certain food, it may actually indicate that your body is low on certain vitamins or minerals. As a result, your body seeks out a certain food that it thinks will provide it with this vitamin or mineral. This reaches your consciousness in the form of an intense craving. In this case, the body is trying to help itself by telling you what to eat. For this reason, understanding your cravings could help you give your body exactly what it is longing for.

For example, if you are craving juice or pop or other sugary drinks like this, consider that you might actually be dehydrated and, therefore, thirsty. Sometimes we see drinks in our fridge, and since we are thirsty, we really want them. Next time you are craving a sugary drink, try having a glass of water first, then wait a few minutes and see if you are still craving that Coca-Cola. You may not want it anymore once your thirst is quenched.

If you are craving meat, you may feel like you want some fried chicken or a hot dog. This can indicate a deficit of iron or protein. The best sources of protein are chicken breast cooked in the oven, and iron is best received from spinach, oysters, or lentils. If you think you may not like these foods, there are many different ways to prepare them, and you can likely find a way that you like.

- Prevents overeating

It can be hard to know how much to eat and when you have had enough to eat without letting yourself eat too much. Sometimes people will eat until the point that they begin to feel completely full. Many times, we keep eating until we become stuffed, even to the point of making ourselves feel physically ill. Intuitive eating will help you to avoid this, as this kind of eating encourages you to give your body what it needs in order to take great care of it. Stuffing your body until it is too full is not what your body is asking for, and once you become accustomed to listening to your body's needs, you will know when it is time to stop.

- Helps you break free from self-judgment

intuitive eating will help you to finally make peace with your body and yourself as a whole. It does this by showing you that your body has needs and that there is no shame in tending to these needs, as long as you do so in a healthy way.

You cannot fully embrace and practice intuitive eating if you have those nagging feelings of self-judgment each time you take a bite of food or decide that you are going to eat lunch when you are hungry. For this reason, in order to practice intuitive eating, you must understand that feeding your body is an act of compassion for yourself and that this does not need to come with self-judgment.

- It is inclusive, not exclusive

One of the great things about this style of eating is that it is not founded on restricting a person's intake of certain foods or allowing only a small variety of foods.

Diets like this are extremely hard to transition to and are hard to maintain for a long period of time. Intuitive eating is about including as many natural whole foods as you wish, while also ensuring that you are consuming enough of all of your nutrients. With this style of eating, you can eat whatever you wish, whenever you wish. This makes it much easier to stick with this type of diet and reduces the chances of falling off after a short period of time due to cravings or intense hunger. It does not restrict calories or reduce your intake greatly, which makes it easier to handle than a traditional diet for many people. It feels natural to eat in this way, which makes it effective.

Chapter 5: Intuitive Eating Part 2

In this chapter, we are going to continue our examination of intuitive eating by looking at some more specific details related to this diet, as well as how to make it a regular part of your life.

How to Make Intuitive Eating Part of Your Life

One of the best ways to make this type of eating a part of your life is to practice it with intention. This is especially important when you are just beginning. Each time you feel a pang of hunger or a compulsion to eat, take a minute to examine your inner world. By doing this, you will get your mind and body accustomed to working together. In addition, do the same after you eat. By doing these two things, you will be able to ensure that you are eating when hungry and stopping when satisfied.

When you finish eating a meal, rank your level of fullness on a scale of 1 to 10, 1 being extremely hungry and 10 being extremely stuffed. This will help you to determine if you are successfully stopping when you are satisfied and not overeating.

It is also important that you learn how to deal with your emotions and feelings in an effective way without using food. Using the techniques that you have learned in this book, you will be able to address your inner demons, which will make space for you to listen to your body and its needs.

As you know by now, listening to your body, your emotions and your mind is extremely important when it comes to practicing intuitive eating. As long as you remember this, you will be well on your way to becoming a lifelong intuitive eater.

What Kind of Foods Should You Choose?

Fish is a great way to get healthy fats into your diet. Certain fish are very low in carbohydrates but high in good fats, making them perfect for a healthy diet. They also contain minerals and vitamins that will be good for your health. Salmon is a great fish to eat, as it is versatile and delicious. Many fish also include essential fatty acids that we can only get through our diet. Other fish that are good for you include:

- Sardines
- Mackerel
- Herring
- Trout
- Albacore Tuna

Meat and Poultry make up a large part of most Americans' diets. Meats and poultry that are fresh and not processed do not include any carbohydrates and contain high levels of protein. Eating lean meats helps to maintain your strength and muscle mass and gives you energy for hours. Grass-fed meats, in particular, are rich in antioxidants.

Eggs are another amazing, protein-filled food. Eggs help your body to feel satiated for longer and also keeps your blood sugar levels consistent, which is great for overall health. The whole egg is good for you, as the yolk is where the nutrients are. The cholesterol found within egg yolks also has been demonstrated to lower your risk of getting diseases like heart diseases, despite what most people think. Therefore, do not be afraid of the egg yolk!

Legumes are a great source of protein as well as fiber, and there are many different types to choose from. These include the following:

- All sorts of beans including black beans, green beans, and kidney beans
- Peas
- Lentils of all colors
- Chickpeas
- Peas

Examples of fruits that you can eat include the following:

- Citrus fruits such as oranges, grapefruits, lemons, and limes
- Melons of a variety of sorts
- Apples
- Bananas
- Berries including strawberries, blueberries, blackberries, raspberries and so on
- Grapes

Vegetables are a great source of energy and nutrients, and they include a wide range of naturally occurring vivid colors which should all be included in your diet.

- Carrots
- Broccoli and cauliflower

- Asparagus
- Kale
- All sorts of peppers including hot peppers, bell peppers
- Tomatoes
- Root vegetables (that are a good source of healthy, complete carbohydrates) such as potatoes, sweet potatoes, all types of squash, and beets.

Seeds are another great source of nutrients, vitamins, and minerals, and they are very versatile. These include the following:

- Sesame seeds
- Pumpkin seeds
- Sunflower seeds
- Hemp, flax and chia seeds are all especially good for your health

Nuts are a great way to get protein if you are choosing not to eat meat or if you are vegan. They also are packed with nutrients. Some examples are below.

- Almonds
- Brazil Nuts
- Cashews
- Macadamia nuts
- Pistachios
- Pecans

There are some **healthy fats** that are essential components of any person's diet, as the beneficial compounds that they contain cannot be made by our bodies; thus, we rely solely on or diet to get them. These compounds are Omega-3 Fatty

Acids, monounsaturated and polyunsaturated fats. Below are some healthy sources of these compounds:

- Avocados
- Healthy, plant-based oils including olive oil and canola oil
- Hemp, chia and flax seeds
- Walnuts

When it comes to carbohydrates, these should be consumed in the form of **whole grains**, as they are high in fiber, which will help to prevent overeating. Whole grains also include essential minerals- those that we can only get from our diet just like those essential compounds found in healthy fats. These essential minerals are selenium, magnesium, and copper. Sources of these whole grains include the following:

- Quinoa
- Rye, Barley, buckwheat
- Whole grain oats
- Brown rice
- Whole grain bread can be hard to find these days in the grocery store, as many brown breads disguise themselves as whole grain when, in fact, they are not. However, there are whole grain breads if you take the time to look at the ingredients list.

Nutrients You Need and How to Get Them

In this section, we are going to look at the most beneficial nutrients for your body and where/ how you can find them. This will help you to decide which foods to include in your diet so that you can ensure you are getting all of the nutrients that your body needs.

1. Omega-3 Fatty Acids

Some vitamins and nutrients are called "essential nutrients." Omega-3 Fatty Acids are an example of this type of nutrient. They are called essential nutrients because they cannot be made by our bodies; thus, they must be eaten in our diets. These fatty acids are a very specific type of fatty acid, and this type, in particular, is the most essential and the most beneficial for our brains and bodies.
They have numerous effects on the brain, including reducing inflammation (which reduces the risk of Alzheimer's) and maintaining and improving mood and cognitive function, including specifically memory. Omega-3's have these greatly beneficial effects because of the way that they act in the brain, which is what makes them so essential to our diets. Omega-3 Fatty Acids increase the production of new nerve cells in the brain by acting specifically on the nerve stem cells within the brain, causing new and healthy nerve cells to be generated.

Omega-3 fatty acids can be found in fish like salmon, sardines, black cod, and herring. It can also be taken as a pill-form supplement for those who do not eat fish or cannot eat enough of it. It can also be taken in the form of a fish oil supplement like krill oil.

Omega-3 is by far the most important nutrient that you need to ensure you are ingesting because of the numerous benefits that come from it, both in the brain and in the rest of the body. While supplements are often a last step when it comes to trying to include something in your diet, for Omega-3's, the benefits are too great to potentially miss by trying to receive all of it from your diet.

Magnesium

Magnesium is beneficial for your diet, as it also helps you to maintain strong bones and teeth. Magnesium and Calcium are most effective when ingested together, as Magnesium helps in the absorption of calcium. It also helps to reduce migraines and is great for calmness and relieving anxiety. Magnesium can be found in leafy green vegetables like kale and spinach, as well as fruits like bananas and raspberries, legumes like beans and chickpeas, vegetables like peas, cabbage, green beans, asparagus, and brussels sprouts, and fish like tuna and salmon.

Calcium

Calcium is beneficial for the healthy circulation of blood, and for maintaining strong bones and teeth. Calcium can come from dairy products like milk, yogurt, and cheese. It can also be found in leafy greens like kale and broccoli and sardines.

Chapter 6: How to Make These New Choices a Habit

Now that you have learned a wealth of information about intuitive eating, we are going to look at some strategies that you can use to make these new, healthy choices a habit. This will take time, but by employing these strategies, you will surely find success.

Healthy Thinking Patterns

In this section, we will look at a real-life example of dealing with challenges to demonstrate healthy thinking patters when it comes to intuitive eating.

Let's say you are trying to focus on healthy eating, and you find that you have had trouble doing so. Maybe you ate a cupcake, or maybe you had a soda at breakfast. From the perspective of traditional diet mentality, this would become a problem for the diet, and this would become a problem in your mind as well. You would likely be beating yourself up and feeling terrible about the choice you have made.

Let's look at this example in more detail. It is very important to avoid beating yourself up or self-judging for falling off the wagon. This may happen sometimes. What we need to do though, is to focus not on the fact that it has happened, but on how we are going to deal with and react to it. There are a variety of reactions that a person may have to this type of situation. We will examine the possible reactions and their pros and cons below:

- You may feel as though your progress is ruined and that you might as well begin again another time. This could lead you to go back to your old ways and keep you from trying again for quite some time. This could happen many times, over and over again, and each time you slip up, you decide that you might as well give up this time and try again, but each time it ends the same.

- You may fall off of your plan and tell yourself that this day is a write-off and that you will begin again the next day. The problem with this method is that continuing the rest of the day as you would have before you decided to make a change will make it so that the next day is like beginning all over again, and it will be very hard to begin again. You may be able to begin again the next day, and it could be fine, but you must be able to really motivate yourself if you are going to do this. Knowing that you have fallen off before makes it so that you may feel down on yourself and feel as though you can't do it, so beginning again the next day is very important.

- The third option, similar to the previous case, you may fall off, but instead of deciding that the day is a write-off, you tell yourself that the entire week is a write-off, and you then decide that you will pick it up again the next week. This will be even harder than starting again the next day as multiple days of eating whatever you like will make it very hard to go back to making the healthy choices again afterward.

- After eating something that you wish you hadn't (and that wasn't a healthy choice), you decide not to eat anything for the rest of the day so that you don't eat too many calories or too much sugar, and decide that the next day you will start over again. This is very difficult on the body as you are going to be quite hungry by the time the evening rolls around. Instead of forgiving yourself, you are punishing yourself, and it will make it very hard not to reach for chips late at night when you are starving and feeling down.

- The fifth and final option is what you should do in this situation.

This option is the best for success and will make it the most likely that you will succeed long-term. If you fall off at lunch, let's say, because you are tired and, in a rush, and you just grab something from a fast-food restaurant instead of going home for lunch or buying something at the grocery store to eat, this is how we will deal with it. Firstly, you will likely feel like you have failed and may feel quite down about having made an unhealthy choice. Now instead of starving for the rest of the day or eating only lettuce for dinner, you will put this slip up at lunch behind you, and you will continue your day as if it never happened. You will eat a healthy dinner as you planned, and you will continue on with the plan. You will not wait until tomorrow to begin again; you will continue as you would if you had made that healthy choice at lunch. The key to staying on track is being able to bounce back. The people who can bounce back mentally are the ones who will be most likely to succeed. You will need to maintain a positive mental state and look forward to the rest of the day and the rest of the week in just the same way as you did before you had a slip-up. One bad meal out of the entire week is not going to ruin all of your progress and recovering from emotional eating is largely a mental game. It is more mental than anything else, so we must not underestimate the role that our mindset plays in our success or failure.

By using this type of thinking, you will set yourself up for success and will not fall off of your plan completely after one slip up.

Healthy Lifestyle Changes

One important way to ensure that these healthy choices stick for good is by changing some aspects of your lifestyle. By doing this, you will reduce the chances of slipping up by eliminating them altogether. For example, you can change the way you approach the grocery store.

When you are entering the grocery store, it is important that you change a few things about the way you shop, in order to set yourself up for success. This is especially important when you are just beginning your intuitive eating practice, as it will be challenging for you to enter the grocery store and avoid cravings and temptations.

The first thing to keep in mind when grocery shopping for a new diet is to enter with a list. By doing this, you are giving yourself a guide to follow, which will prevent you from picking up things that you are craving or things that you feel like eating in that moment.

One of the biggest things to keep in mind when beginning a new eating practice like intuitive eating is to avoid shopping when you are hungry. This will make you reach for anything and everything that you see. By entering the grocery store when you are satiated or when you have just eaten, you will be able to stick to your list and avoid falling prey to temptations.

If you treat your grocery shopping experience like a treasure hunt, you will be able to cross things off of the list one at a time without venturing to the parts of the grocery store that will prove to be a challenge for you to resist. If you are making healthy eating choices, you will likely be spending most of your time at the perimeter of the grocery store. This is where the whole, plant-based foods are located. By doing this, and entering with a list, you will be able to avoid the middle aisles where the processed, high-sugar temptation foods are all kept.

Having a plan is key when it comes to succeeding in learning new habits and employing a new lifestyle. This plan can be as detailed as you wish, or it can simply come in the form of a general overview. I recommend you start with a more detailed plan in the beginning as you ease into things.

As everyone is different, you may be the type of person who likes lots of lists and plans, or you may be the type of person who doesn't, but for everyone, beginning with a plan and following it closely for the first little while is best. For example, this plan can include things like what you will focus on each week, what you will reduce your intake of, and what you will try to achieve in terms of the mental work involved.

Once you have come up with a general plan for your new lifestyle and how you want it to look, you can then begin laying out more specific plans.

Planning your individual meals will make it much easier for you when you get home from work or when you wake up tired in the morning and need to pack something for your lunch.

You can plan your meals out a week in advance, two weeks or even a month if you wish. You can post this up on your fridge, and each day you will know exactly what you are eating, with no thinking required. This way, there won't be a chance for you to consider ordering a pizza or heating up some chicken fingers because you will already know exactly what you are going to make. By approaching your new style of eating in this way, you can make this transition easier on yourself and ensure success every step of the way.

30-Day Meal Plan

The following 30-day meal plan includes a variety of meals that you can make in order to keep your first thirty days interesting and tasty!

Day 1

- Breakfast:

Coffee

Feta, mushroom and spinach, omelet.

- Lunch:

Oven-baked tempeh with broccoli and cauliflower rice.

- Dinner:

Chicken Caesar salad- tofu and romaine lettuce, parmesan

Day 2

- Breakfast:

Unsweetened yogurt with a mix of some berries such as strawberries, raspberries, and some seeds like flax seeds and chia seeds, and nuts like sliced almonds and walnuts.

- Lunch:

A healthy lunch-time salad with avocado, cheese, grape tomatoes, and a variety of nuts and seeds like spicy pumpkin seeds. Add a salad dressing on top such as blue cheese or ranch dressing, or a homemade one using olive oil and garlic.

- Dinner:

Chicken breast with onions and a homemade tomato sauce. Served alongside some grilled zucchini or eggplant.

Day 3

- Breakfast:

A no sugar added full fat Greek yogurt bowl with seeds, nuts and berries.

1 Cup of coffee

- Lunch:

Make your own lunch box, including firm tofu or meat of some sort, raw tomatoes, any type of cheese cubes that you wish, pickles, a hard-boiled egg, vegetables such as celery, carrots, radishes or zucchini, nuts for protein and fat such as walnuts, or almonds, homemade guacamole (avocado, onion, garlic, jalapeno).

- Dinner:

Grilled portobello, grilled eggplant and grilled zucchini as well as cherry tomatoes sautéed in extra virgin olive oil with garlic. Served with rice and protein such as pork or chicken.

Day 4

- Breakfast:

Coffee

Homemade mushroom & Spinach Frittata, including any vegetables that you wish such as bell peppers and onion.

- Lunch:

Cream cheese with cucumber slices for dipping.

Hard-boiled egg

Meatballs with sweet and sour sauce

- Dinner

Bacon, Avocado, Lettuce, Tomato panini.

Day 5

- Breakfast:

Egg Salad with lettuce, cucumber and whole grain bread.

- Lunch:

Homemade guacamole (avocado, onion, garlic, jalapeno, lime juice) with raw zucchini slices for dipping.

Hard-boiled egg

Tuna

- Dinner:

Cauliflower gratin (cheese, cauliflower, onion, garlic and so on)

As well as chopped lettuce drizzled with Caesar Dressing

Day 6

- Breakfast:

Coffee with heavy cream or coconut oil.

Celery sticks, dipped in peanut or Almond Butter

- Lunch:

Leftover cauliflower gratin

As well as chopped lettuce drizzled with Caesar Dressing

- Dinner:

Cooked or raw broccoli with grated cheese on top

Steak seared in olive oil

Day 7

- Breakfast:

Pancakes with fresh fruits

Black Coffee

- Lunch:

Cold pasta salad with fresh vegetables

Feta and Tomato Meatballs

Raw fresh spinach

- Dinner:

Spicy Spaghetti Squash Casserole

Fresh spinach, raw or cooked with 1 Tbsp ranch dressing drizzled on top.

Day 8

- Breakfast

Smoothie

- Lunch

Tempeh meatballs with guacamole and raw vegetable salad

- Dinner

Rice noodle stir fry with your choice of vegetables and tofu

Day 9

- Breakfast

Omelet cooked in coconut oil with cheese, onions, bell pepper and tomatoes

- Lunch

Tofu scramble with vegetables such as spinach and mushrooms and cheese

- Dinner

Curry with chicken, rice and coconut milk sauce with hot chili paste

Day 10

- Breakfast

Full fat yogurt unsweetened with berries, chia seeds, flax seeds

- Lunch

Cobb salad with boiled egg, vegetables of your choice, tofu, tempeh or chicken and Caesar dressing

- Dinner

Homemade pizza with your choice of toppings

Day 11

- Breakfast

Smoothie with chia seeds and flax seeds, berries and plant-based protein powder, as well as plant-based milk

- Lunch

Salad with tofu or boiled egg, olive oil dressing, spinach and diced vegetables

- Dinner

Vegetarian frittata using coconut oil, spinach, mushroom, cheese, bell peppers and tomato

Day 12

- Breakfast

Greek yogurt no sugar added with nuts and seeds

- Lunch

Homemade tacos with your choice of toppings, including ground turkey

- Dinner

Macaroni and cheese with crumbled roasted bread crumbs on top

Day 13

- Breakfast

Whole grain oats with no sugar added, nuts, flax and chia seeds as well as heavy cream and a plant-based nut butter.

- Lunch

Lettuce wraps with curried tofu and grilled eggplant and zucchini

- Dinner

Homemade burritos filled with crumbled, seasoned meat of your choice, sour cream, guacamole and diced tomatoes

Day 14

- Breakfast

Greek yogurt no sugar added with nuts and seeds

- Lunch

Avocado egg bowls with bacon

- Dinner

Fried rice with your choice of vegetables, scrambled egg and tofu

Day 15

- Breakfast

Coffee with heavy cream and no sugar added

- Lunch

Carrots with guacamole, cottage cheese with nuts and seeds and homemade baked zucchini chips with olive oil drizzle

- Dinner

Egg Salad with Lettuce Wraps

Day 16

- Breakfast

Pancakes with no sugar added maple syrup

- Lunch

Vegetarian egg quiche with spinach and mushroom

- Dinner

Broccoli salad with onion, a cheese of your choice, creamy ranch dressing, almonds and walnuts sliced, as well as some avocado and tofu cubes

Day 17

- Breakfast

Potato hash browns fried in olive oil, sunny side up egg and tempeh "bacon" with a side of grilled tomatoes

- Lunch

Avocadoes stuffed with cauliflower "taco meat", homemade salsa with tomatoes and herbs, sour cream, and grated cheese

- Dinner

Cooked or raw broccoli

Small amount of butter that can be added to the broccoli for taste

Grated cheese on top that can also be added to the broccoli

With steak seared in olive oil

Day 18

- Breakfast

Shakshuka with eggs, tomatoes and parsley

- Lunch

Grilled zucchini roll ups with tomato and cheese

- Dinner

Coconut milk curry with rice, bell peppers and tofu

Day 19

- Breakfast

Breakfast smoothie with berries, no sugar added and full fat milk

- Lunch

Broccoli and cheese fritters with homemade hummus to dip and a side of carrots, celery and cucumber for dipping

- Dinner

Cobb salad including hard-boiled egg, ham cubes, your choice of vegetables and an olive oil or ranch dressing

Day 20

- Breakfast

Spinach and mushroom frittata

- Lunch

Sandwich with scrambled eggs, spinach and mushrooms cooked in olive oil and topped with lettuce, tomato or any other fillings or toppings you wish to include. Finally, add a homemade creamy avocado sauce with avocado, cilantro, pepper and salt and some sour cream.

- Dinner

Rice risotto with cheese, vegetable broth and mushrooms

Day 21

- Breakfast

Unsweetened yogurt with a mix of berries such as strawberries, raspberries, and some seeds like flax seeds and chia seeds, and nuts like sliced almonds and walnuts.

- Lunch

Caesar salad- dressing with no sugar added

Raw vegetables, mixed greens and tempeh

- Dinner

Cauliflower gratin- cheese, cauliflower and choice of vegetables

Day 22

- Breakfast

Hash browns fried in olive oil, sunny side up egg and bacon with a side of grilled tomatoes

- Lunch

Stuffed half zucchini with feta cheese, tomato sauce (no sugar added) and herbs for topping

- Dinner

Mashed potatoes using whole milk and cheese, with grilled eggplant and mushrooms

Day 23

- Breakfast

Nut butter smoothie with yogurt, nut butter, flax seeds, chia seeds

- Lunch

Pan fried steak seasoned with herbs and olive oil, paired with

A spinach salad with raw vegetables of choice and no sugar added Caesar dressing

- Dinner

Cauliflower pasta salad with celery, spinach, onions, and walnuts

Day 24

- Breakfast

Feta, mushroom and Spinach, omelet

Coffee

- Lunch

Coleslaw with a creamy cilantro dressing, carrots, cabbage, celery, tomato and herbs for topping

- Dinner

Crispy tofu cubes with zucchini noodles and a homemade peanut sauce

Day 25

- Breakfast

No bake protein bars

Coffee with no sugar added

- Lunch

Roasted tomatoes with goat cheese, spinach, cilantro and olive oil & balsamic drizzle

- Dinner

Eggplant and zucchini "French fries" with olive oil and crispy tofu cubes

Baked chicken breast

Day 26

- Breakfast

Pancakes with no sugar added maple syrup, full fat Greek yogurt and berries for topping

- Lunch

Low carb broccoli cheese soup with crispy cauliflower on the side

- Dinner

Curried rice with choice of vegetables, such as bell peppers and broccoli

Day 27

- Breakfast

Breakfast salad with scrambled egg, avocado, mixed greens, grilled tomatoes and cheese

- Lunch

Fried goat cheese with roasted red peppers, spinach and olive oil drizzle

- Dinner

Spicy Spaghetti Squash Casserole

Fresh spinach, raw or cooked with ranch dressing drizzled on top

Day 28

- Breakfast

Full fat yogurt unsweetened with berries, chia seeds, flax seeds

- Lunch

Vegetarian chili with tomato, sour cream, a variety of beans and tomatoes

- Dinner

Zucchini spiral pasta noodles with creamy yogurt avocado sauce

Day 29

- Breakfast

Cauliflower "bread" grilled cheese sandwich (similar to cauliflower crust pizza but made as a grilled cheese sandwich instead.

- Lunch

Green beans with mushrooms and tomatoes with a chicken breast on the side

- Dinner

Grape tomato marinara on pasta noodles with parmigiano Reggiano cheese and fresh cracked pepper.

Day 30

- Breakfast

Egg taco shells filled with choice of vegetables

- Lunch

Baked crispy tofu steaks with a sesame seed crust on a bed of zucchini strips and spinach

- Dinner

Baked Spaghetti squash filled with roasted tomatoes and eggplant, topped with melted, crispy cheese

Chapter 7: What to Do Next

As you take all of this information forth with you, it may seem overwhelming to begin applying this to your own life. Remember, life is a process, and you do not need to expect perfection from yourself right away. By taking the first step-reading this book, you are already on your way to changing your life. If you fall off and find that you are back to your old ways, try to find inspiration in the pages of this book once again. If you find that you are unable to find success on your own, there is no shame in seeking professional help. There are many people who are trained professionals in dealing with disordered eating and who can serve as a mentor or a guide for you as you navigate this challenge.

How To Seek Help If It Becomes Uncontrollable?

Understanding and accepting that you need help is the first step to recovery. By reading this book, you have taken this step. If you need further help, there is no shame in accepting this fact. There are many ways to seek help for disordered eating, depending on the level of help that you need. Below is a list of ways that you can seek help, ordered from least to most help.

- Online resources
- Support System
- Support Group
- Group counseling
- Anonymous online counseling or telephone counseling
- One on One counseling

- Talk therapy
- Rehab centers

Counseling or Therapy

Talking therapies are very effective treatments for disordered eating. The things that people learn in therapy gives them the insight and skills in order to feel better and tackle their eating disorder, as well as to prevent it from coming back in the future.

One example of talk therapy is Cognitive Behavioral Therapy or CBT. The way that cognitive behavioral therapy works is by putting an emphasis on the relationship between a person's thoughts, emotions, and behaviors. The theory behind this is that when a person changes any one of these components, change will be initiated in the others. The goal of CBT is to help a person decrease negative thoughts or the amount of worry they experience in order to increase their overall quality of life.

If you think that this is something you would benefit from, please reach out to your local resources to find out more.

PART IV

You will find many of the Chinese recipes will call for shoyu. Shoyu is the term broadly given to soy sauces that are made from fermented soybeans, wheat, salt, and water. In general, they are quite thin and clear and are excellent as an all-purpose cooking and table sauce. One of the best selling shoyu in the world is proclaimed to be Kikkoman Soy Sauce.

Chapter 1: Soup

Hot & Sour Soup

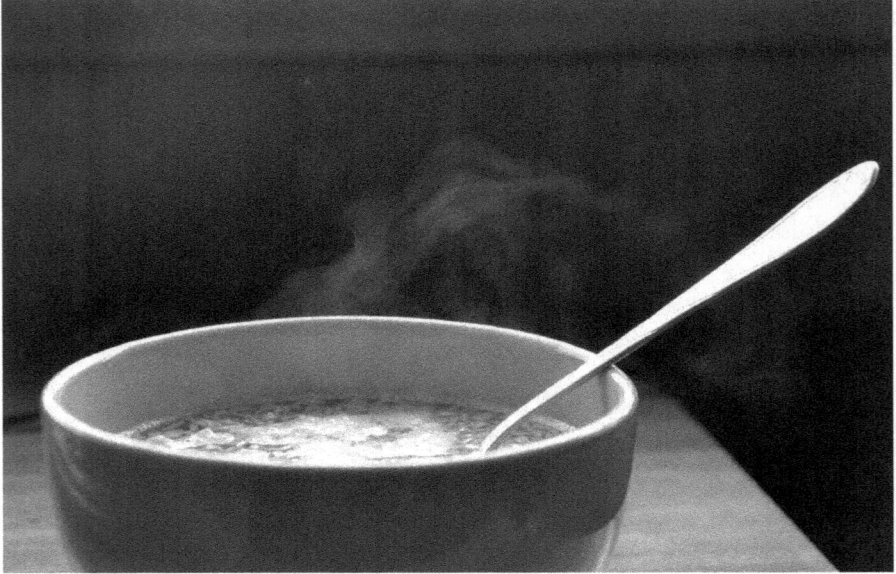

Servings Provided: 4

Time Required: 40 minutes

What is Needed:

- Chicken broth - low-sodium (1 quart)
- Dried tree ear fungus (.25 cup)
- Dried lily buds (12)
- Medium-dark soy sauce (2 tbsp. + more for seasoning)
- Distilled white vinegar (2 tbsp. + more for seasoning)
- Cornstarch (2 tbsp.)
- Kosher salt (.5 tsp.)
- Large eggs (2)

- Bamboo shoots (.5 cup - shredded)
- Cooked pork, ham, or chicken (.5 cup - shredded)
- Spiced thick - dry tofu - shredded (1 cup/3.5 oz.)
- White pepper - finely ground (1.5 tsp.)
- Sesame oil (1 tbsp.)
- To serve: Chopped cilantro & scallions

Preparation Method:

1. Dump the lily buds into boiling water to soak about ten minutes until they're softened. Discard the rough tips.

2. Prepare another container and add the tree fungus and boiling water to soak from 20 minutes to half an hour. Rinse, drain, and coarsely chop them.

3. Dump the broth into a large saucepan. Once boiling, add the soy sauce, salt, and vinegar.

4. Whisk three tablespoons of water with the cornstarch and mix it into the broth to simmer for three to four minutes to thicken.

5. Once it's at a rolling boil, whisk the eggs and a dash of salt, and work it into the soup in a circular fashion. Wait five seconds, stir and extinguish the heat.

6. Toss in the tofu, chicken, white pepper, bamboo shoots, ear fungus, and lily buds.

7. Simmer the soup using the medium temperature setting for about two minutes, adding in vinegar, soy sauce, and salt as desired.

8. Portion the soup and garnish it using the cilantro, scallions, and a spritz of sesame oil.

Wonton Soup

Servings Provided: 8

Time Required: 1 hour 15 minutes

What is Needed:

- Pork - fresh loin - whole (.5 lb.)
- Crustaceans - shrimp - mixed-species - raw (2 oz.)
- Brown sugar (1 tsp.)
- Burgundy wine (1 tbsp.)
- Shoyu - low-sodium soy sauce (1 tbsp.)
- Spring onions/scallions - tops & bulb (1 tsp.)
- Ginger root (1 tsp.)
- Wonton wrappers - includes egg roll wrappers (24 @ 3.5-inch square)
- Clear chicken broth - Swanson - CAM (3 cups)
- Scallions (includes tops and bulb- (1/8 cup)

Preparation Method:

1. Chop the green onion and add one teaspoon into a large mixing container and add the pork, shrimp, sugar, wine, shoyu sauce, and ginger. Thoroughly toss the mixture and let stand for 25 to 30 minutes.
2. Scoop the filling (1 tsp.) into the middle of each wonton skin.

3. Moisten the four edges of the wonton wrapper with a small amount of water on your fingertips, and pull the top corner down to the bottom, folding the wrapper over the filling to create a triangle.

4. Seal it by pressing the edges firmly. Bring the left and right corners together above the filling and overlap the corner of the tips. Moisten with water and press together. Repeat the process until all wrappers are used.

5. Make the soup. Heat the chicken stock to a rolling boil. Add the wontons and cook for five minutes.

6. Top off the soup with chopped green onions and serve.

Chapter 2: Seafood

Honey Walnut Shrimp

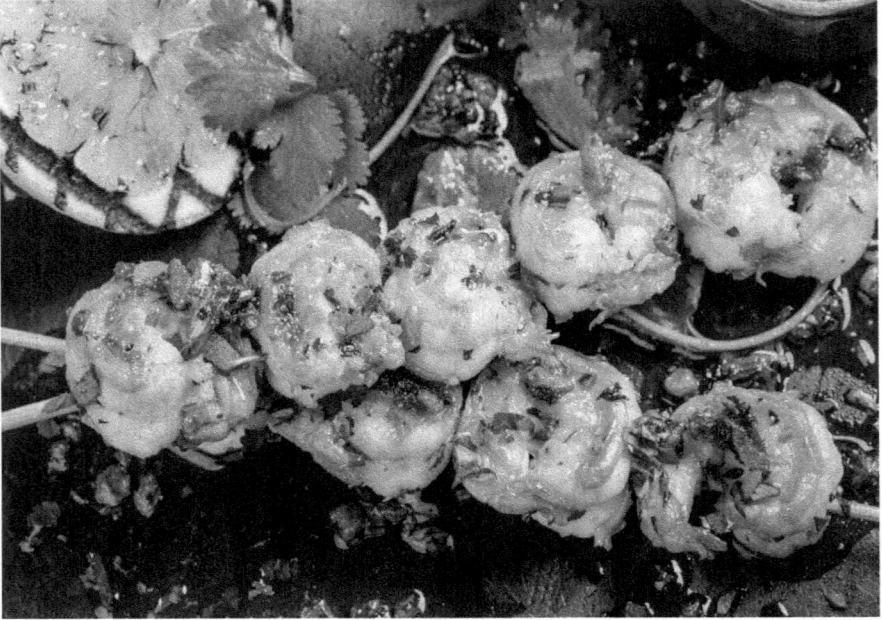

Servings Provided: 4

Time Required: 30 minutes

What is Needed:

- Water (1 cup)
- English walnuts (.5 cup)
- Granulated sugar (2/3 cup)

- Egg white - raw (4)
- Rice flour - white (2/3 cup)
- Salad dressing/soybean oil with salt/mayonnaise (.25 cup)
- Jumbo shrimp - fresh & raw (1 lb./21-30)
- Honey - strained or extracted (2 tbsp.)
- Sweet condensed canned milk (1 tbsp.)
- Oil for frying (1 cup)

Preparation Method:

1. Whisk the water and sugar in a small saucepan. Once boiling, add the walnuts and boil them for two minutes. Dump them into a colander to drain. Arrange the nuts on a baking tray to thoroughly dry.
2. Whip the egg whites in a mixing container until they're foamy. Stir in the mochiko until it's a pasty consistency.
3. Warm the oil using the med-high temperature setting in a heavy deep skillet.
4. Dip the shrimp into the batter, and fry them until nicely browned (5 min.). Transfer them to a paper towel-lined platter using a slotted spoon to allow them to drain.
5. Whisk the honey, mayonnaise, and sweetened condensed milk. Fold in the shrimp and toss to coat with the sauce.
6. Garnish using the candied walnuts right before serving.

Steamed Fish

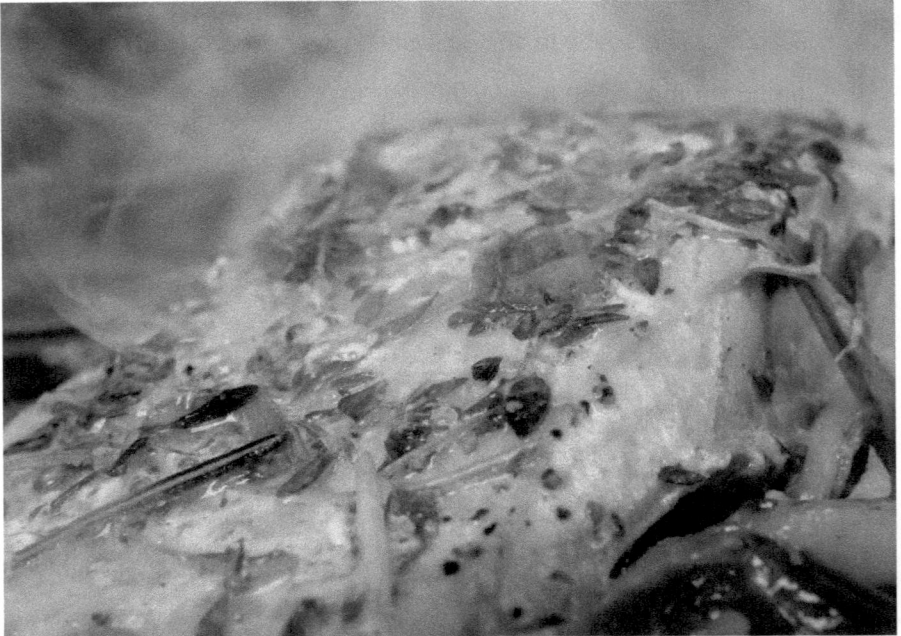

Servings Provided: 2

Time Required: 35 minutes

What is Needed:

- Raw finfish, snapper, mixed species (1 lb.)
- Salt (.5 tsp.)
- Black pepper (.5 tsp.)
- Ginger root - raw (1 tbsp.)
- Shoyu soy sauce (1 tbsp.)
- Sesame oil (2 tsp.)

- Shiitake mushrooms - raw AMM (2)
- Tomatoes (1 fresh)
- Peppers - raw red-hot chile (half of 1)
- Cilantro (2 sprigs - raw)

Preparation Method:

1. Prepare a steamer with a basket large enough for the snapper to lie flat. Pour in 1.5 inches of water and wait for it to boil.
2. Sprinkle the snapper with pepper and salt and pepper before placing it into the basket. Top the fish with ginger, and drizzle with sesame oil and soy sauce.
3. Place the tomatoes, mushrooms, and red chile pepper in the steamer basket.
4. Set a timer and steam the fish for 15 minutes, or until easily flaked with a fork. Garnish with cilantro and serve.

Stir-Fried Shrimp & Scallions

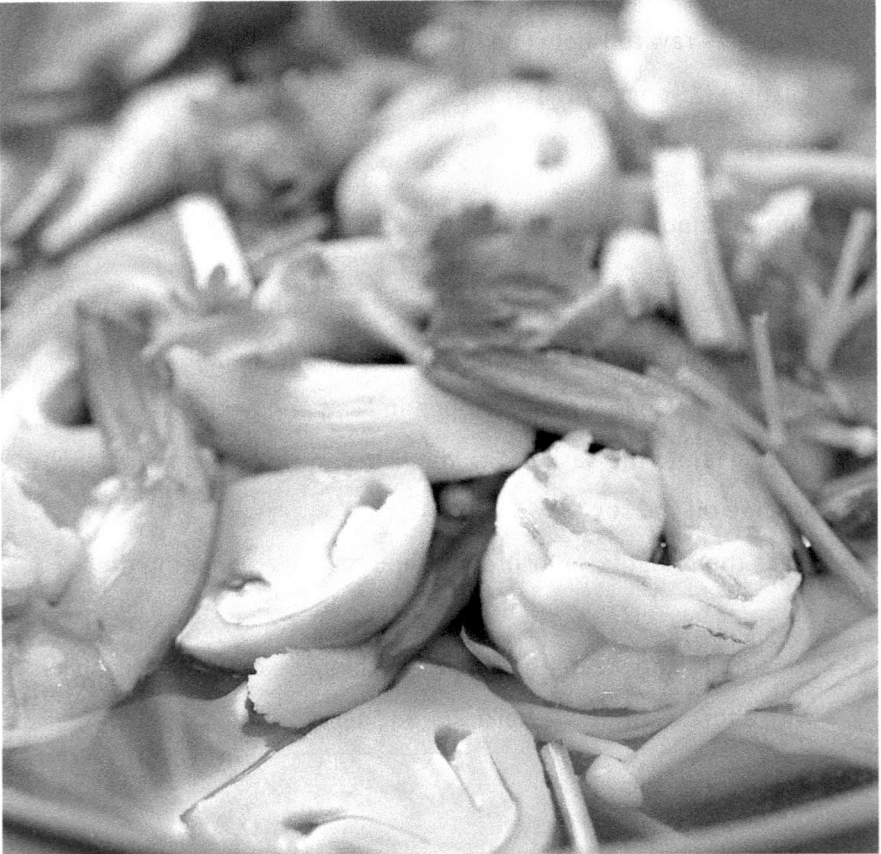

Servings Provided: 4

Time Required: 30 minutes

What is Needed:

- Jumbo shrimp (1.5 lb.)
- Garlic (3 cloves)

- Fresh ginger (1-inch section)
- Crushed red pepper (1.5 tsp.)
- Egg white (1 large)
- Cornstarch (2 tsp. - divided)
- Ketchup (.75 cup)
- Chicken broth - low-sodium (.5 cup)
- Black pepper & kosher salt (1.5 tsp. each)
- Sugar (1 tbsp.)
- Canola oil (.25 cup)
- Chopped cilantro (.5 cup)
- Scallions (3)

Preparation Method:

1. Thinly slice the scallions. Shell and devein the shrimp. Mince the garlic and ginger.
2. Toss the shrimp with the ginger, garlic, red pepper, one teaspoon of the cornstarch, and egg white until well-coated.
3. Whisk the broth with the ketchup, sugar, salt, and pepper with the rest of the cornstarch.
4. Warm a large skillet with the oil until it shimmers. Add the shrimp and stir-fry using the high-temperature setting until pink.
5. Add the ketchup mixture and simmer until the shrimp are heated (2 min.). Stir in the cilantro and scallions to serve.

Chapter 3: Poultry

Kung Pao Chicken - Keto-Friendly

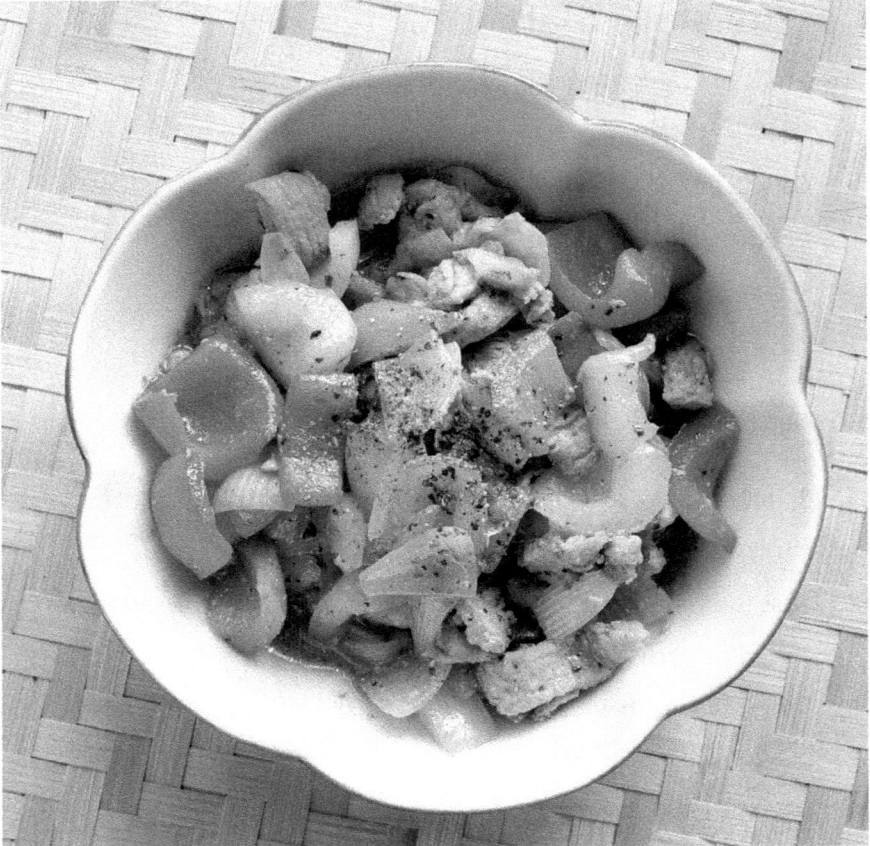

Servings Provided: 4

Time Required: 40 minutes

What is Needed:

- Chicken breasts - boneless skinless (1 lb.)

  The Marinade:

- Chinese rice wine/dry sherry (2 tsp.)
- Soy sauce (2 tsp.)
- Cornstarch (2 tsp.)

  To Cook:

- Olive oil or sunflower oil (3 tbsp. divided)
- Dried red chilies (4-6)
- Green onions (4)
- Optional: Red finger chili (1)
- Asparagus (1 bunch)
- Sweet bell pepper (1)
- Garlic & ginger (4 tsp. each)
- Mini cucumbers (2)
- Roasted salted peanuts/cashews (.33 cup)
- Toasted sesame seeds (1 tsp.)

  The Sauce:

- Water (3 tbsp. - cold)
- Soy sauce & white vinegar (2 tbsp. each)
- Chinese wine/ sherry (1 tbsp.)
- Cornstarch (2 tsp.)
- Salt (.5 tsp.)
- Optional: Asian chili-garlic sauce (1 tbsp.)

Preparation Method:

1. Slice the chicken into one-inch chunks and combine it with the marinade fixings in the first group (soy sauce, rice wine, and

cornstarch) stirring to combine. Marinate the mixture for 15 minutes.

2. Prep the veggies by cutting the asparagus into large pieces and mincing the garlic and onion. Chop the cucumber. Core and cube the bell pepper. Cut the green onions into one-inch pieces.

3. Prepare a large-sized cast-iron pan to warm one tablespoon of oil using the med-high temperature setting. Add the green onions, dried chilies, and finger chili.

4. Simmer the mixture until the green onions are slightly charred (1 min.). Transfer them to a baking sheet or large platter.

5. Heat the rest of the oil in the pan (1 tbsp.). Add asparagus and bell pepper and cook, stirring until it's slightly charred (2-3 min.).

6. Transfer to a baking tray and add the remainder of the oil (1.5 tsp.) to the pan. Working in two batches, stir-fry the chicken until browned (3-4 min. per batch), repeating with remaining oil.

7. Make the Sauce: Whisk the water, rice wine, soy sauce, and cornstarch until smooth. Return the chicken, vegetables, and chilies to the pan.

8. Sprinkle with salt, stir in the sauce, and cook until the liquid is bubbling and thickened (30 seconds to one minute). Stir in the cucumbers, peanuts, and chili-garlic sauce.

9. Serve it with a garnish of sesame seeds.

Orange Chicken

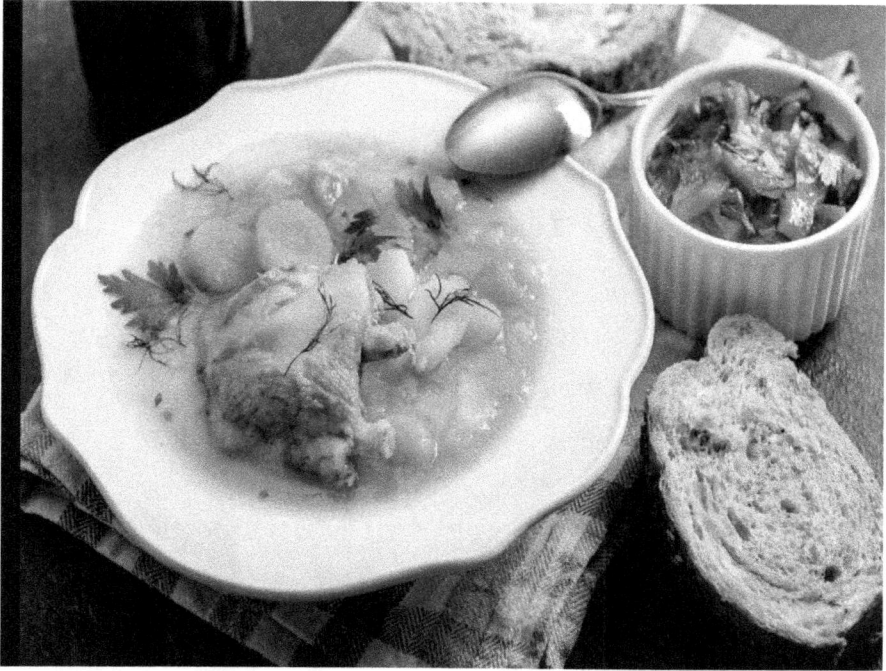

Servings Provided: 4

Time Required: 35 minutes

What is Needed:

The Chicken:

- Oil (as needed for frying)
- Boneless & skinless chicken breasts (4)
- Eggs (3 whisked)
- Cornstarch (.33 cup)

- Flour (.33 cup)

Orange Chicken Sauce:

- Orange juice (1 cup)
- Sugar (.5 cup)
- Rice/white vinegar (2 tbsp.)
- Tamari or soy sauce (2 tbsp.)
- Ginger (.25 tsp.)
- Garlic powder (.25 tsp.) or 2 garlic cloves (2 finely diced)
- Red chili flakes (.5 tsp.)
- Orange Zest (1 orange)
- Cornstarch (1 tbsp.)

The Garnish:

- Orange Zest
- Green Onions

Preparation Method:

1. Prepare the orange sauce. Mince the ginger and garlic. Pour the vinegar, orange juice, soy sauce, sugar, garlic, ginger, and red chili flakes into a saucepan. Sauté them for about three minutes.
2. Whisk one tablespoon of cornstarch with two tablespoons of water to form a paste. Add it to the orange sauce and whisk thoroughly. Continue cooking the sauce for about five minutes, until the mixture begins to thicken. After it's thickened, remove the pan from the burner and add the orange zest.

3. Prepare the chicken by cutting it into bite-sized chunks.

4. Dump the flour, a pinch of salt, and cornstarch in a pie plate or another shallow dish.

5. Whisk eggs in a shallow mixing container.

6. Dip the pieces of chicken into the egg mix and then flour mixture. Place them onto a platter.

7. Next, warm two to three inches of oil in a heavy-bottomed skillet (med-high temperature). Use an electric skillet or use a thermometer to check the heat until it reaches 350° Fahrenheit.

8. Working in batches, fry several chicken pieces at a time. Cook them for two to three minutes, often turning until golden brown, and place the chicken on a paper-towel-lined plate. Repeat the process until all the chicken is cooked.

9. Toss the chicken with the orange sauce. Reserve some of the sauce to serve over the rice. Serve it with a sprinkling of green onion and orange zest to your liking.

Chapter 4: Pork

Chinese Pork BBQ (Char Siu)

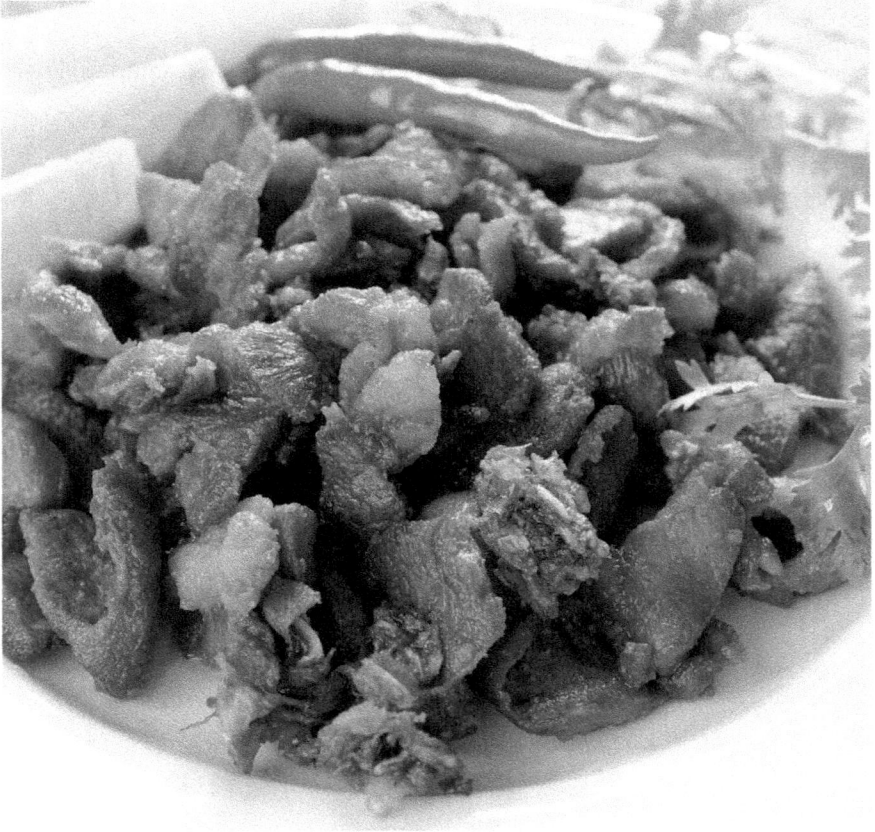

Servings Provided: 4

Time Required: 3 hours 40 minutes

What is Needed:

- Fresh pork tenderloin - lean cut (2 lb.)
- Soy sauce -shoyu - made from soy and wheat (.5 cup)
- Honey - strained/extracted (.33 cup)
- Ketchup (.33 cup)
- Brown sugar (.33 cup)
- Hoisin sauce - ready-to-serve (2 tbsp.)
- Rice wine (.25 cup)
- Red food coloring (.5 tsp.)
- Chinese Five-Spice Powder (1 tsp.)

Preparation Method:

1. Cut the pork "with the grain" into strips 1.5-2-inches long, and toss it into a large resealable zipper-type baggie.
2. Whisk the soy sauce, ketchup, honey, hoisin sauce, brown sugar, red food coloring, Chinese 5-spice, and rice wine in a saucepan using the med-low temperature setting. Simmer it until just combined and slightly warm (2-3 min.). Pour the marinade into the bag with the pork, pushing the air from the bag, and zip it closed. Toss the bag several times to cover all pork pieces.
3. Pop the pork in the fridge for two hours or overnight.
4. Warm the outdoor grill using the med-high temperature setting and lightly grease the grate.
5. Transfer the pork from marinade, shaking it to remove excess juices. Discard the marinade.
6. Grill the pork for 20 minutes. Place a container of water onto the grill and continue cooking, turning the pork until cooked thoroughly or about one hour. It's ready when the internal temp reaches 145°

Fahrenheit.

Chinese Pork Dumplings

Servings Provided: 5/50 dumplings

Time Required: 1 hour 20 minutes

What is Needed:

- Soy sauce made from wheat & soy - shoyu (.5 cup)
- White rice vinegar CBT (1 tbsp.)
- Chinese chive - kucai - raw (1 tbsp.)
- Dried sesame seeds - whole (1 tbsp.)
- Sriracha sauce/Chili puree sauce w/Garlic CBT (1 tsp.)
- Freshly ground pork - raw (1 lb.)
- Garlic (3 cloves)
- Egg - whole (1)
- Kucai - Chinese chive - raw (2 tbsp.)

Preparation Method:

1. Combine ½ cup of the soy sauce, rice vinegar, sesame seeds, one tablespoon of chives, and the chile sauce in a small mixing container. Set it to the side for now.

2. Mix the pork, minced garlic, egg, two tablespoons of chives, soy sauce, sesame oil, and ginger in a large mixing container until thoroughly combined.

3. Lightly flour a workspace. Place a dumpling wrapper onto it and spoon about one tablespoon of the filling in the center.

4. Wet the edge with a little water and crimp it together, forming small pleats to seal the dumpling. Repeat the process with the rest of the dumpling wrappers and filling.

5. Warm one to two tablespoons of oil in a large skillet using the med-high temperature setting. Arrange eight to ten dumplings in the pan and cook until browned (2 min. per side).

6. Pour in one cup of water, place a lid on the pot, and simmer until the pork is thoroughly cooked and the dumplings are tender (5 min.).

7. Continue the process until all dumplings are prepared. Serve with the soy sauce mixture for dipping.

Chop Suey

Servings Provided: 6

Time Required: 51 minutes

What is Needed:

- Fresh pork tenderloin (1 lb.)
- Wheat flour, all-purpose, white, enriched, bleached (.25 cup)
- Oil - soybean, salad or cooking (2 tbsp.)
- Bok choy - raw (2 cups)
- Celery - fresh (1 cup)
- Sweet red bell peppers (1 cup)
- Mushrooms (1 cup)
- Water chestnuts, Chinese, canned - solids & liquids (8 oz. can)
- Garlic (2 fresh cloves)
- Swanson Clear Chicken Broth CAM (.25 cup)
- Shoyu sauce (.25 cup)
- Cornstarch (1 tbsp.)
- Fleischmann's Cooking Sherry II (1 tbsp.)
- Ground ginger (.5 tsp.)

Preparation Method:

1. Use a sharp knife to discard the fat from the pork and slice it into one-inch pieces. Combine the flour and pork in a resealable bag, seal, and shake it thoroughly to cover.

2. Warm one tablespoon oil in a large skillet using the med-high heat setting. Add the trimmed pork and cook for three minutes or until browned. Transfer it to a container and keep it warm.

3. Pour the rest of the oil in the pan to heat. Add the celery, bok choy, mushrooms, red pepper, garlic, and water chestnuts. Stir-fry them for three minutes.

4. Thoroughly whisk the chicken broth, soy sauce, cornstarch, sherry, and ginger in a mixing container.

5. Combine the pork and broth mixture in a skillet, and cook for one minute or until thickened.

Easy Moo Shu Pork

Servings Provided: 6

Time Required: 1 hour 20 minutes

What is Needed:

- *Shoyu* - Soy sauce made from soy + wheat (2 tbsp.)
- Sesame oil (1 tbsp.)
- Garlic (1 tsp.)
- Fresh ginger root (1 tbsp.)
- Pork tenderloin (.75 lb.)
- Oil - soybean - salad or cooking (2 tbsp.)
- Chinese cabbage (pe-tsai) (2 cups)
- Carrots (1 raw)
- Salt (1 pinch)

Preparation Method:

1. Whisk the sesame oil, soy sauce, garlic and ginger in a bowl until the marinade is smooth. Dump it into a resealable plastic bag and add the pork. Cover it using the marinade, squeeze out any excess air, and seal the bag. Marinate in the fridge for a minimum of one hour to overnight.

2. Warm vegetable oil in a wok/large skillet using the medium temperature setting. Rinse and add the cabbage and diced carrot. Simmer the mixture for one to two minutes.

3. Push the cabbage mixture aside and add pork with marinade to the center of the skillet. Cook and stir until the pork is thoroughly cooked (3-4 min.).

4. Scoot the cabbage into the center of the skillet and continue to cook it for another minute or two. Adjust the flavor with a portion of pepper and salt to your liking.

Peking Pork Chops - Slow-Cooked

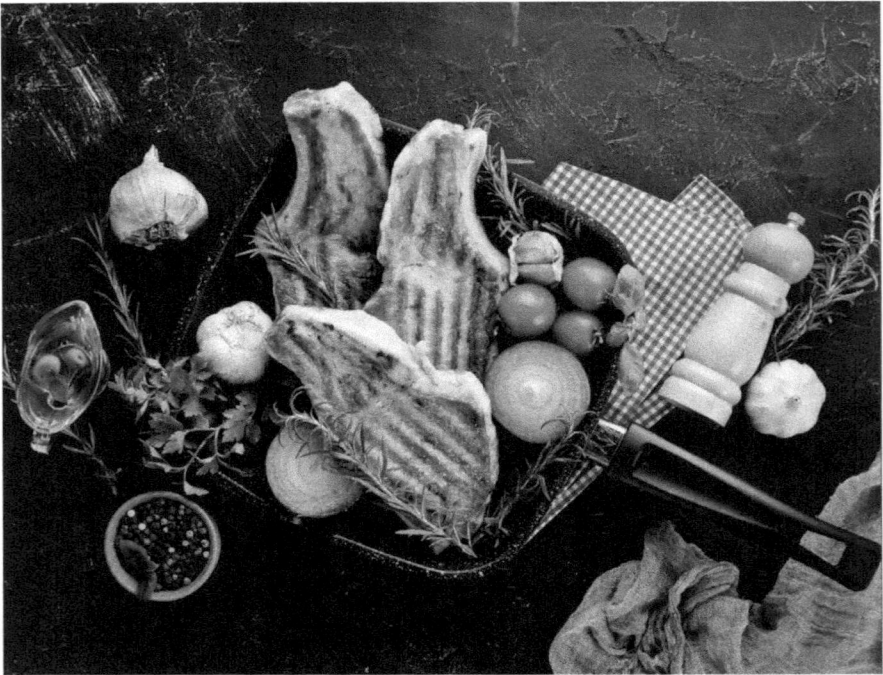

Servings Provided: 6

Time Required: 6 hours 15 minutes

What is Needed:

- Pork chops - top loin (6 boneless)
- Brown sugars (.25 cup)

- Ground ginger (1 tsp.)
- Shoyu soy sauce (.5 cup)
- Ketchup (.25 cup)
- Garlic (1 clove)
- Salt (as desired)

Preparation Method:

1. Use a sharp knife to remove the fat from the chops and toss them into the cooker.
2. Whisk the sugar, soy sauce, ginger, garlic, pepper, and salt. Dump it over the meat
3. Securely close the lid and set the timer for four to six hours.
4. Serve when it's tender with a dusting of salt and pepper as desired.

Chapter 5: Other Chinese Dishes

Crispy Tofu With Sweet & Sour Sauce

Servings Provided: 4

Time Required: 45 minutes

What is Needed:

The Sauce:

- Cornstarch (2 tsp.) + Water (2 tsp.)
- Garlic (2 minced cloves)
- Freshly grated ginger (.5 tsp.)
- Chili pepper flakes (.25 tsp.)
- Vegetable oil (2 tsp.)
- Water (.5 cup)
- Unseasoned rice vinegar (.33 cup)
- Agave nectar (.5 cup)
- Low-sodium soy sauce (2 tbsp.)
- Tomato paste (2 tbsp.)
- Sea salt (.25 tsp.)

   The Tofu & Batter:

- Medium/firm tofu (1 brick)

- For Frying: Vegetable oil (3 cups)
- Cornstarch (1 tbsp.)
- Brown rice flour (1 cup)
- Ground pepper (.25 tsp.)
- Sea salt (.5 tsp.)
- Garlic powder (.5 tsp.)
- Cold soda water (1 cup)

Preparation Method:

1. Drain the brick of tofu and chop it into bite-sized cubes. Continue to drain the cubes on a layer of paper towels to remove the excess water. Press it often while you prepare the sauce.
2. Mix water with the cornstarch in a cup and set it aside for now.
3. Warm two teaspoons of vegetable oil using the med-low temperature setting. Mince and add the ginger, garlic, and chili pepper flakes. Stir for 30 seconds to one minute until fragrant.
4. Whisk in the rest of the sauce ingredients using the medium setting until it's bubbly. Whisk in the cornstarch mixture.
5. Whisk the sauce often for 10-12 minutes until slightly thickened. Transfer the pan to a cool burner while you prepare the crispy tofu.
6. Warm three cups of oil in an electric skillet or pan to reach 375° Fahrenheit.
7. Mix the batter by combining the rice flour, cornstarch, sea salt, garlic powder, and ground pepper in a mixing container.
8. When the pan is hot, stir in the soda water to the flour mixture and

mix well.

9. Use your hands to coat three to four cubes of tofu and gently place them into the oil. Fry them for 2-2.5 minutes.

10. Remove the tofu using a slotted spoon and place them onto a layer of paper towels to absorb the excess fat. Repeat the process with the rest of the tofu cubes.

11. Warm the sauce if needed. In two to three batches, you can coat the crispy tofu with sauce by adding a portion of the sauce to a large bowl and tossing the crispy tofu cubes until coated evenly. Serve to your liking with veggies or rice.

Shiitake & Scallion Lo Mein

Servings Provided: 8

Time Required: 40 minutes

What is Needed:

- Lo mein noodles (1 lb.)
- Snow peas (.25 lb.)
- Mirin (.25 cup)
- Soy sauce (.25 cup)
- Toasted sesame oil (2 tsp.)
- Canola oil (3 tbsp.)
- Shiitake mushrooms (1 lb.)
- Scallions (6)
- Fresh ginger (1 tbsp.)
- Water (2 tbsp.)
- Cilantro (2 tbsp.)

Preparation Method:

1. Slice the snow peas diagonally into halves. Remove the stems and thinly slice the caps of the mushrooms. Cut the scallions into one-inch lengths. Mince the ginger and chop the cilantro.

2. Prepare a large pot of boiling salted water. Cook the noodles until tender, adding in the snow peas for the last two minutes of the cooking cycle. Rinse and drain the noodles and snow peas in a colander using cold water until cooled.

3. Whisk the soy sauce with the sesame oil and mirin.

4. Prep a deep skillet to warm two tablespoons of the canola oil until shimmering using the high-temperature setting. Add the shiitake and cook it, undisturbed, until browned (5 min.).

5. Add the rest of the canola oil, scallions, and ginger. Stir-fry until the scallions softened (3 min.).

6. Add the water into the pan and simmer using moderate heat, scraping up the browned bits from the bottom of the pan for about a minute or so.

7. Mix in the snow peas, noodles, and soy sauce mixture. Simmer while tossing the noodles until they are thoroughly heated (2 min.).

8. Sprinkle using the cilantro and transfer it onto banana leaf cones or bowls to serve.